Praise for Disaster Mental Health books by George W. Doherty

"Mr. Doherty has produced an invaluable reference volume for everyone involved in disaster response/disaster preparedness field. It is a must for your library! His attention to detail, breadth of scope, depth of knowledge and readable writing style, reflect the work of an eminent scholar in his field and one who has paid his dues on the frontlines. It represents the ultimate A to Z 'How to Do It' manual in this difficult, complicated field. From the sensitive discussion of clinical issues to the organizational planning details, the clarity and thoroughness of this volume are outstanding. This book should be required reading for everyone involved in this critical field."

John G. Jones, Ph.D. ABPP ATR-BC Licensed Psychologist

"Disasters happen—and someone has to be there to help the victims. George W. Doherty discusses training practices for mental health professional whose task it is to assist victims of disaster-related stress and trauma, giving advice and tips about dealing with various disasters whether they be the product of man or nature. His books are recommended to anyone whose career may take them into this type of profession and for any community library social science shelf."

—*Midwest Library Review*

"As a certified first responder with the City of Austin Emergency Measures Office I was delighted to find more information to add to my training. (The City of Austin provided training as a result of 9/11 in the event Austin, Texas, experiences a disaster from terrorists or other incidents of major concern.) George W. Doherty's book certainly presents a concise and informative addition to the library of a first responder, either beginner or one that is experienced. The information is well-researched and appropriate. Furthermore, I believe his books could be used by trainers when creating first responder to disaster training courses and be part of the study material."

—Irene Watson, Managing Editor, *Reader Views*

"This is an information-packed book about disasters and crises, the psychological impact of such events upon people, from the victims to the disaster workers, and also a psychological explanation of those who create crises, such as terrorists. Anyone who is considering being a disaster worker of any type, whether it is working for an organization like FEMA or even being an EMT, police officer, or volunteer fireman will find value in this book as it lays out various situations and what the disaster worker should know and be prepared to handle since an emergency or crisis could happen unexpectedly at any time."

—Tyler R. Tichelaar, PhD

"Awareness of how crises affect various people-groups, thinking through the important role disaster workers play in re-establishing normalcy in people's shaken lives, and planning immediate and long-term approaches to help traumatized people recapture mental equilibrium are vital aspects of a crisis intervention program. This is a beneficial and informative tool to raise awareness and plan levelheaded crisis intervention."

—Michael Philliber, PhD, for *Rebeccas Reads*

"It is extremely important for health practitioners and emergency workers to be prepared for emergencies, natural disasters, terroristic attacks and times of war. When dealing with traumatic incidents such as these, everyone is affected, including the victim, their family members and health care professionals. By being prepared to deal with these issues, research has shown that early intervention can reduce the chances of PTSD, acute anxiety, and depression. Ways to be prepared for these situations are discussed and a variety of other factors are identified that can increase the likelihood that disorders will occur. Having an operational emergency plan prepared ahead of time can make a huge difference in the ability to be prepared for the crisis.

"I found *Return to Equilibrium* to be very informative and necessary for mental health practitioners. As a person who works with disabled students in the community college setting, I also believe that this information is pertinent to college counselors and instructors. The better our understanding, the better we can serve their needs and help them reestablish equilibrium."

—Paige Lovitt, for *Reader Views*

Crisis in the American Heartland:

Disasters & Mental Health in Rural Environments

Introduction (Volume 1)

George W. Doherty, MS, LPC

Foreword by Thomas Mitchell, MS LPC

Crisis in the American Heartland: Disasters & Mental Health in Rural Environments
An Introduction (Volume 1)

Library of Congress Cataloging-in-Publication Data

Doherty, George W. (George William)
Crisis in the American heartland : disasters & mental health in rural environments / George W. Doherty.
    v. ; cm.
Includes bibliographical references and index.
Contents: v. 1. Introduction
ISBN-13: 978-1-61599-075-7 (pbk. : alk. paper)
ISBN-10: 1-61599-075-5 (pbk. : alk. paper)
ISBN-13: 978-1-61599-076-4 (hardcover : alk. paper)
ISBN-10: 1-61599-076-3 (hardcover : alk. paper)
 1. Crisis intervention (Mental health services)--United States. 2. Emergency management--United States. 3. Psychiatric emergencies--United States. I. Title.
 [DNLM: 1. Crisis Intervention--United States. 2. Disaster Planning--United States. 3. Emergency Services, Psychiatric--United States. 4. Rural Health--United States. WM 401]
 RC480.6.D639 2011
 362.2'1--dc22
                          2011000004

The Rocky Mountain Region Disaster Mental Health Institute is a 501(c)3 Non-profit Organization. Learn more at www.RMRInstitute.org

Rocky Mountain DMH Institute Press is an Imprint of:
Loving Healing Press Inc.   www.LHPress.com
5145 Pontiac Trail   info@LHPress.com
Ann Arbor, MI 48105   Tollfree 888-761-6268
USA   Fax +1 734 663 6861

Contents

Objectives

Following completion of this course, you should be able to:

- Describe how disasters affect people in rural environments.
- Identify, explain and discuss cross-cultural considerations in rural environments.
- Describe mental health services provided by mental health professionals in rural areas.
- Identify how rural communities work together to prepare for response and recovery from critical incidents, crises, and disasters.
- Identify and describe the background and factors affecting farm and ranching crises.
- Describe and explain the factors affecting and causing stress on farms and ranches in the western US and other rural environments.
- Describe and identify stress, anxiety, and cross-cultural variables in rural areas.
- Identify problems associated with trauma situations in rural areas.
- Describe cultural competency and its importance in rural environments.
- Identify special populations present in rural areas.
- Explain the importance of rural culture, ethnicity and cultural values in responding to critical incidents, crises and disasters in rural populations.
- Explain how rural practice differs from urban environments.
- Describe mental health approaches to disasters in rural environments.
- Identify types of disasters and their impacts that affect rural areas.
- Identify and describe the phases of disaster and how they affect rural areas.

- Identify and describe support networks and resources in rural environments available for disaster responses.
- Identify and describe symptoms of psychological trauma.
- Explain BASIC-ID and how this multi-modal approach is used to help identify areas of concern for assessment following disaster and critical incident traumas.
- Identify and describe the challenges associated with mental health responses in rural areas and how to meet them.
- Identify and describe the roles of country doctors and rural mental health professionals and paraprofessionals.

Foreword

When I wandered out into the high plains of eastern Wyoming as a newly minted mental health professional, I experienced a period of culture shock. Many of the services needed for individuals and families were often not available in the rural area I worked and, when available, would often be underutilized. People in the farming and ranching communities had their own way of dealing with the vicissitudes of life and were more likely to "cowboy up" than take steps to resolve problems or seek help when needed.

After a few years, my employer sent me out to obtain some training in disaster mental health. I met George Doherty at a training held on the campus of the University of Wyoming. The result for me was fortuitous as not only did I have access to training resources through George's Rocky Mountain Region Disaster Mental Health Institute, but the added opportunity to learn a few things about rural mental health and how to better serve Wyoming's rural and agricultural-oriented population. George has been a practitioner in rural settings for more years than he prefers to acknowledge and has developed many insights into serving rural populations.

Rural people across the world are both similar to and very different from their urban neighbors. Oftentimes the realities of rural living create a need to develop skills in self-sufficiency that, when combined with an attitude of "rugged individualism," can make it difficult for rural individuals to reach out for help when warranted. Resources are fewer and often geographically separated by hundreds of miles. Crises in rural settings may not be newsworthy to the extent that a similar crisis in an urban setting would be. As a result the extent of a disaster might not become apparent for many days. Any response requiring human services and material supports can be delayed, and hampered by minimal or absent infrastructure, further hampering recovery efforts.

George's *Crisis in the American Heartland: Disasters & Mental Health in Rural Environments* was written for a broad audience of planners, health and mental health professionals. The following chapters summarize the character of rural residents and the challenges of rural living, rural economy, challenges of rural life, and a number of hazards or disasters that have or can occur in rural settings. Georges devotes a section to review the unique vulnerabilities to stress as well as the impact of crisis in rural settings. He includes brief reviews of the components of Critical Incident Stress Management. He concludes with a section on preparation for crisis and assembling appropriate staff for the occasions when a concerted response to crisis is needed.

Thomas Mitchell, MS LPC
Peak Wellness Center
Torrington, Wyoming

1   Introduction to Crises in Rural Areas: Background and Overview

A review of the current literature reveals a number of published studies and articles that deal with a broad cross-section of topics on crisis intervention and related areas (CISM, Trauma, Disaster) in rural environments. These include CISM services in rural settings (Seebold, 2003); Telehealth services (Dimmick, Burgiss, Robbins, Black, Jarnagin & Anders, 2003); stress in rural areas (Cowen, 2001); suicide intervention (Aoun & Johnson, 2001); rural elderly (Neese, Abraham, & Buckwalter, 1999; Snustad, Thompson-Heisterman, Neese & Abraham, 1993); responses in rural communities following natural disasters (Sundet & Mermelstein, 1996); community action for abusive men (Hanson & Whitman, 1995); litigation in rural practice (Bushy & Rauh, 1993); rural crisis intervention teams (Silver & Goldstein, 1992); childhood depression (Cecchini, 1998); rural psychiatry in hospital emergency rooms (Morris, 1997); intervention with at-risk adolescents (Rose-Gold, 1991); Guidance in small schools (Dinkmeyer, 1990); cultural aspects (Paulsen, 1988a; Paulsen, 1988b); responses of rural ministers to natural disasters (Echterling, Bradfield, Wylie, 1988); the farm crisis (Mermelstein, 1987; Thompson & McCubbin, 1987; Hargrove, 1986); rural sexual abuse prevention (Johnson, 1987); short-term interventions with families and children following tornadoes (McRee, Corder, Deitz, Silverstein, et al., 1985-1986); disasters in small communities (Farberow, 1985); crisis intervention in rural schools (Wise & Smead, 1985; Harper, 1984; Beare, 1981); rural psychiatric training (Bassuk & Cote, 1983); use of paraprofessionals in rural populations (Shybut, 1982; Marshall, 1971); working with rural families (Anderson, 1976); and approaches to drug prevention and treatment in rural areas (Bourne, 1974). A literature search revealed a total of 37 articles published on these topics since 1974. While this is probably not inclusive of all the work done on crisis intervention in rural areas, it does suggest a lack of dissemination of such information to mental health and related professionals.

Paulsen (1988) discussed the economic crisis affecting rural America in terms of its impact on the individual and his or her community. She outlined three themes: (1) rural communities are in a state of chronic crisis, (2) rural individuals are members of a distinctly unique culture, and (3) the rural crisis warrants a unique response from mental health professionals. All three of these provide insights into rural crises and all three deserve further study.

Harper (1984) discussed crisis intervention and management techniques in rural or remote areas, focusing on rural Alaska, and suggested guidelines for successful interventions which highlighted the importance of understanding cultural differences. These are important considerations in most rural areas in the United States as rural areas tend to follow cultural traditions more than urban areas, in general.

Telephone crisis lines are one method that has been used in both rural and urban areas. Shybut (1978) found that underutilization, especially by males and by the elderly of both sexes, was the initial problem on a crisis intervention telephone service used in a rural area. Telecounseling and other forms of counseling, including online counseling on the internet, are areas that present potential for covering large geographic areas common in the rural west.

Over the past 20 years, there has been a crisis in many farming communities as the face of agriculture in the country has changed. Many family farms were lost or sold with attendant stressors on those involved. Hargrove (1986) examined the myth of rural communities uniting under stress, and suggests clinical and community activities for mental health workers during farm crises. In his article, he maintained that a model for understanding human response to natural disasters is useful for understanding response to such crises. He offered recommendations at the community level and suggested that the clinical/advocate model developed by G. B. Melton (1983; see also PA, Vol. 61: 9256) provides a useful perspective from which to operate.

Farm and Ranching Crises

Treatment approaches to such crises vary. For example, Jurich & Russell (1987) evaluated 15 farm families that underwent therapy at the Kansas State University

Family Center, using a model of family adaptation to stress developed by H. I. McCubbin et al. (see record 1981-30250-001). Major interventions included reframing, mobilizing resources, and utilizing less indirect means of intervention. Subjects (Ss) showed a greater increase in well-being at three months than did a general sample of clients. However, stress levels were not lowered as much as the general sample, and life satisfaction was lower at follow-up than the general population. Thompson & McCubbin (1987) outline some resource materials available to help educators, counselors, and others to support rural families in crises and to facilitate decision making, long-range planning, and problem solving. Counseling programs, workshops, publications, support groups for coping with for stress, and computerized decision aids are reviewed.

In another approach, Paulsen (1988) asserts that rural crises create new numbers of rural individuals who are in need of assistance as they cope with the stress of economic dislocation and the overwhelming difficulties that occur after the loss of a farm or business. She discusses individual, family, and community treatment aspects within the thematic context of a culture in crisis. An urban-based regional family service agency, Farmers Helping Farmers, is presented as an example of a systems response to the rural crisis. The proposed treatment involves a multilevel community response that includes self-help support groups, instruction of adaptive coping skills, and sharing information in rural communities. Mental health professionals are challenged to further their understanding of rural crises and to adopt more flexible treatment strategies to encompass a multilevel system's response.

In the current times of crisis, nationally and internationally, with increased levels of stress, anxiety, and concern about terrorism, it is critical that mental health professionals in rural areas become aware of recent research, training and approaches to crisis intervention, traumatology, compassion fatigue, disaster mental health, critical incident stress management, post-traumatic stress, and related areas.

Waterfield (1986) covered the growing economic and cultural split between rural and urban America. In his book *Conflict and Crises in Rural America*, he addressed many of the major issues impacting rural areas. These include such issues as: the "rural-urban wars" over land use, control of water, cheap food policy, trade, the use of chemicals and pesticides, animal rights, the biases in urban-dominated media, corruption in food marketing and distribution, what is happening to the land, and who the largest landowners are. Waterfield suggests that rural America's share of national wealth is declining and that America is the world's best hope for solving the problems of hunger and rural poverty.

Through a long-term (1982-1989) study of 156 farm families in Dodge County, Georgia, Barlett (1993) discusses the damage from a decade of crisis, and provides a critical look at trends in American farming, their impact on rural community vitality, and the effects of federal farm legislation. This was a study of family farms in Dodge County, Georgia. It examined the social and economic factors that determine success in farming today. Bartlett, a professor of anthropology at Emory University, presents an agrarian history of Dodge County and its changes and transformations from frontier times through the present. The key period of her study was the boom-and-bust decade of the 1980's when the nation was in the grip of a farm crisis.

Using data derived from interviews and personal observations of 124 small and medium-scale farm families, Bartlett describes in detail the coping strategies and management approaches of those who were determined to stay in farming and those who left. She explores family histories, personal aspirations, and attitudes about farming as a livelihood. Her interviews with farm women reveal a variety of role definitions and spousal relationships that enable farm families to remain intact. The aftermath of the crisis and its impacts on farm size, resource conservation, and management style offer insights for family farm survival in other communities.

Rural psychology has very few major studies concerning practice in rural environments and small communities. Practitioners face some very different problems from their more urban counterparts. Rural practice presents important yet challenging issues for psychology, especially given the North American and international distribution of the population, levels of need for psychological services in rural settings, limited availability of rural services, and migration of rural residents to urban centers. Direct service issues include the need to accommodate a wide variety of mental health difficulties, issues related to client privacy and boundaries, and practical challenges. Indirect service issues include the greater need for diverse professional activities, including collaborative work with professionals having different orientations and beliefs, program development and evaluation, and conducting research with few mentors or peer collaborators. Professional training and development issues include lack of specialized relevant courses and placements, and such personal issues as limited opportunities for recreation and culture, and lack of privacy. Psychology will need to address more fully these complex issues if rural residents are to receive equitable treatment and services (Barbopoulos & Clark, 2003).

Recent concerns in agriculture have caused people to take a look at where their food comes from. The crisis in the cattle industry as a result of concerns surrounding Mad Cow Disease and, in the Far East, concerns about "Bird Flu" in chickens contribute to stressors not only in the general public, but also among farmers and ranchers who strive to keep the population fed.

The US farm crisis in the 1980s refocused national attention on the plight of rural areas. Data indicate that, relative to urban areas, rural America suffers from the double burden of (a) high levels of poverty, disability, and impairment, and (b) inadequate health and human services. Wagenfeld (1988) introduced a special issue of the *Journal of Rural Community Psychology* that presented a status report on the mental health problems in rural areas during that period. Topics discussed included the social ecology of inpatient mental health services, the response of community mental health centers to the farm crisis, innovative mental health services, policy approaches to improving mental health services, and a research agenda for rural community psychology.

Ramirez-Ferrero (2002) challenges interpretations of the ongoing restructuring of the American agricultural sector as simply an economic phenomenon with psychological consequences. Ramirez-Ferrero argues that male farmers' responses to the farms' financial crisis are not strictly psychological, individual, or idiosyncratic, but cultural. Subjects' actions and beliefs are a consequence of a multiplicity of cultural discourses. It is their socially-constructed sense of self or subjectivity (mediated by cultural processes of power) that determines which ones they internalize, consider, and act upon. Rural northwest Oklahoma served as the locus of this study. Research was conducted with farm families and included the collection of life histories from 13 couples, periodic participant-observation on a farm, unstructured and structured interviews with health professionals, and focus group research. This study incorporated farmers' life stories, particularly those of crisis, to understand local notions of gender, kinship, land, farming styles, familial and farm goals, and community. Informants' life stories are presented in the context of broader discussions of the history of northwest Oklahoma, agricultural economics, corporate, and capitalist processes, and Christianity to understand the social construction of the emotion of pride, an emotion that is critical in understanding men's responses to the farm crisis. Ramirez-Ferrero suggests that emotions are culturally mediated, embodied thoughts that are necessarily evaluative, and therefore challenges the common understanding of emotions as biological and psychological phenomena. Because the patriarchal foundation of farming communities is being eroded by industrial values, men experience the devaluation of cultural ideas that supported their subjectivity, specifically, the emotion of pride. This devaluation, in turn, leads men to actions and inactions that are often negative, destructive, and tragic.

Stein (1984) explored the cultural ethos and psychodynamics underlying a duality in the Midwestern/Southwestern US male character, which is encapsulated in the image of the steadfastly, sedentary farmer and that of the adventuresome vagabond cowboy—both at war with one another in the same person. This duality is considered primarily within the context of Oklahoma's wheat-farming and cattle-ranching families, but it is in fact a variation upon a regional Midwestern / Southwestern US identity. Stein argues that the psychologically primitive qualities attributed and allocated to the Midwest/Southwest by the larger national group keep the unstable regional masculine character "stirred up" and, thereby, available to the rest of the nation as both negative example and positive source for the current national nostalgia, and as support for political "conservatism" and international militarism.

As things change in rural areas, the need for appropriate social services also changes. Martinez-Brawley & Blundall (1991) interviewed 44 farm families in Iowa and Pennsylvania concerning beliefs and attitudes about need and social services. Families in Iowa had been severely affected by an agricultural crisis and were more likely to have had contact with organized social services. Seeking assistance appeared more acceptable in Iowa than in Pennsylvania. Among the families, there was a sense that success and failure had little to do with deservingness. The perception that the world is unfair was overwhelming in Iowa. Families did not view themselves as needing special help as a class of people; yet they did voice concerns about not being understood by outside systems. Services that were found to be the least acceptable in both Iowa and Pennsylvania were those closely associated with depression indicators (e.g. problems with spouse, increased dependency on school, feelings of anxiety or isolation).

Schulman & Armstrong (1990) analyzed interview data from statewide surveys of 670 farm operators, collected during a period of economic and ecological crisis, to examine relationships among perceived stress, social support, and survival in agriculture. While the level of perceived stress had no relationship with survival, social support had a significant impact on both social psychological and behavioral dimensions of survival in agriculture. Perceived social support increased plans to remain in agriculture and increased the probability of a person continuing farming.

Using data from a statewide survey of 725 North Carolina that farm operators collected during a period of economic and ecological crisis in 1986, Schulman & Armstrong (1989) analyzed the relationships between perceived social psychological distress, social support, and demographic, farm structure, and socioeconomic characteristics. Younger operators showed higher distress levels, and age and social support interacted so that social support lowered distress levels more for younger than for older operators. Results also suggested that total family income had a curvilinear relationship with perceived distress. Low and high income farm operators manifested higher levels of distress than middle income operators. Results have implications for policy intervention and farm crisis support programs.

Cook, John R. & Tyler (1989) examined the attitudes of 34 North Dakota farm couples toward receiving help for a personal problem. Statistical significances (Ss) were assigned to groups according to the level of financial coping with respect to the possible loss of their farm (stable, declining, and out of business). Ss who were out of business or declining were more open to receiving help from educational sources than Ss whose farms were stable. Female Ss were open to receiving help regardless of their level of financial coping while their husbands were as receptive to help only at times of financial crisis. Ss showed reluctance in making use of outside resources of any kind.

Leaving the Farm or Ranch

Early on, Lamarche (1960) suggested that rural crises are created by the movement to the city, especially on the part of the young, and abandonment of the land. Rapid social evolution without any preparation can have undesirable psychological effects.

In the 1980s, there was a high level of interest in retirement of farmers because of an aging farm population and concern that the "farm crisis" may have disrupted succession patterns. Keating & Munro (1989) described the process of exit from farm businesses of a group of older farmers and determined the relationship between goals of family succession and behaviors in the exit phase. A sequence of exit from work, management, and ownership was found. Farmers (aged 50+ yrs), who value continuity, were most likely to involve sons in management of the operation. Keating & Munro suggested that programs for two-generation farm families may be useful in the early part of the exit phase while estate planning information and programs may be more appropriate to those in the latter part of the process.

Stress on the Farm and on the Range

Carson, Araquistain, & Ide (1994) examined the relationship between potential family vulnerability factors (stressors and strains), manifestations of maladaptation (family discord and distress), family strengths (hardiness), and measures of bonadaptation (quality of life) as reported by 188 men and women representing 100 Idaho farm and ranch families. Ss completed a battery of tests, including the Farm/Ranch Stress Scale, a demographic questionnaire, and four measures from the Family Invulnerability Test. Family strains and stressors unique to farming and ranching were positively associated with family discord and distress but negatively associated with hardiness and quality of life. Greater family hardiness, as reported by both wives and husbands, was positively correlated with their perceptions of family's quality of life.

Plunkett, Henry , & Knaub (1999) studied 77 adolescents in farm and ranch families to examine the relationship of demographic variables, family stressor events, and family coping strategies to adolescent adaptation. Results indicated that adolescent age and family transitions were positively related to individual stress. Males reported less family stress than did females. Seeking spiritual support was negatively related to family stress, while the perceived impact of the farm crisis was positively related to family stress. Family support was positively related, and family substance use issues were negatively related, to adolescent satisfaction with family life.

Swisher, Elder, & Lorenz (1998) examined how the occupation of farming structures the stress experiences of individuals through the timing and placement of actions. They showed how occupations have effects that spillover into family and friendship relationships. The sample came from the Iowa Youth and Families Project, a longitudinal study of siblings and parents in the aftermath of the farm crisis of the 1980s, and included 424 married couples who had one child in the 7th grade and another child within four years of age of the first child. Results show that farming affects both exposure and vulnerability to stressors. Specifically, farm men are more exposed to financial and job-related stressors, while less prone to marital conflict, than non-farmers. Given the importance of cohesion in farm family operations, farm men are more vulnerable to such conflict when it occurs. However, farm men are unaffected, if not consoled, by knowledge of undesirable events in the lives of their friends. It was concluded that farm men use downward social comparisons to cope with the high levels of uncertainty characteristic of farming in the aftermath of the 1980s' farm crisis. The lives of rural families who suffered economic hardship and economic pressure caused many to face difficult choices in response to hardship. Multiple adjustments created significant pain for many of these families. This was evidenced by the extreme emotional distress among families who lost a farm as a result of the crisis.

Rettig, Danes, & Bauer (1991) describes a resource exchange theory that outlines the dimensions of life quality and presents a multidimensional scale measure of personal evaluations of family life quality based on this theory. The scale includes items representing love, status, services, information, goods, and money resources received from the family. It is suggested that receipt of these resources satisfied personal needs for (1) love and affection, (2) respect and esteem, (3) comfort and assistance, (4) shared meaning, (5) personal things, and (6) money for personal use.

Van Hook (1990) interviewed 49 adolescents (mean age 16.8 yrs) during the farm crisis. In 66% of the families, there was an increase in parental work responsibilities outside the family farm or business. Family tensions increased in response to the economic uncertainties and change in family roles. The farm crisis was an anxious time for Ss, who described major gaps in family and community information systems. Feelings of personal responsibility for family economic problems were found in 63% of the Ss. The determination of Ss to prepare to cope with an uncertain and unfair world may involve the shift from farming to other occupations. Increased levels of anxiety, depression, and suicide attempts make this a high-risk population during difficult times.

Cecil (1998) describes the development and implementation of *Stress: Country Style*, an Illinois program designed as a response to stress problems among farm families created by an economic downturn. The program involved a crisis line, outreach counseling, and community education about stress. The relationship between the program and community mental health centers is also addressed. Successes and failures of the program are considered.

Walker & Walker (1998) studied the self-reported incidence of stress-related symptoms in 476 male and 341 female farmers, and 70 male and 39 female urban residents. Close to 50% of the farmers reported the frequent to constant occurrence of the symptoms of trouble relaxing, loss of temper, and fatigue; over 30% reported similar occurrence rates for 6 additional symptoms. Self-reported symptom rates were significantly higher in farm women than in farm men, higher in younger farmers, higher in mixed farming operations, and higher in farmers who were holding off-farm employment. Symptom scores were significantly higher in the farmers compared with the urban Ss. Scores on five symptoms distinguished farm and urban Ss. Walker & Walker suggest that the chronic stress associated with the farm financial crisis may have caused a high self-reported incidence of symptoms among farmers.

Loeb & Dvorak (1987) discuss the high level of stress experienced by many of today's farm families. They suggest that health professionals should be aware of the current situation to deal effectively with the farm family as a unit. Therapists must be well-versed in farm family dynamics before they can understand the impact of external factors. The following topics are of importance: the economics of farming, the farm family (husband, wife, in-laws, adult children), communication in farm families, and health issues. Loeb & Dvorak conclude that there is no end in sight to the farm crisis and that many more families will need support from trained experts in the future.

Hargrove (1986) examined the myth of rural communities uniting under stress and suggests clinical and community activities for mental health workers during farm crises. A model for understanding human reaction to natural disasters is useful for understanding response, recovery and community cohesiveness following such crises. Hargrove suggests that the clinical/advocate model developed by G. B. Melton (1983; see also PA, Vol. 61:9256) provides a useful perspective from which to operate.

Olson & Schellenberg (1986) examined stressors in farm environments, using data from questionnaire surveys of general, familial, and extrafamilial farm stressors. General stressors include problems such as machinery breakdown and harvests, while familial stressors involve role incongruence and conflict. The discussion of extra-familial stressors emphasizes financial stressors and farm financial crises. Olson & Schellenberg suggest that financial stressors are becoming more intense relative to familial factors because of farm crises. They consider directions for community psychology in terms of four types of programs aimed at preventing or alleviating farm financial stress:

- General education/socialization
- Individual skill training
- Development of supportive social agencies
- Political action

They also note the importance of a multiple program approach emphasizing early detection of farm financial stress.

Farmer (1986) suggests that farmers who have failed in the farm crisis of the 1980s blame themselves, although even top producers and managers had been affected. The prevalence of depression is not surprising considering the severity of the losses, the prolonged nature of the stress, and the minimal control farmers have in overcoming their problems. Participation in farm support groups may be effective for families working through a fairly predictable grief cycle involving denial, anxiety, guilt, anger, hostility, confusion, and depression.

Internal and external threats could soon squeeze some ranch and farm families out of business. To assist ranch families with these threats and with amiably transferring the operation to the next generation, Zimmerman (1984) offers a six-step Consensus Management Model that combines strategic planning with psychoeducation/family therapy. A pilot test with an intergenerational ranch family indicated improvements in family functioning, including reduced stress and depression, and improved self-esteem and family coping levels.

Mental Health, Stress, Anxiety, and Cross-Cultural Variables in Rural Areas of the Western United States

There has been increasing interest worldwide in recent years in the development of comprehensive mental health programs. In a pluralistic society like the United States, successful intervention will quite often depend on how well the therapist knows and understands the client's cultural or ethnic group. Rural areas of the western United States add still another dimension with sometimes large geographical areas populated with diverse ethnic and cultural groups.

The American west has been portrayed in song, story, speech, myth, legend, and films. From the classic tales of Mark Twain to the legends of Butch Cassidy to Native Americans to films about western women, schoolmarms, and prostitutes to the major epic dramas of United States history, the American west has held a fascination for people from many cultures. The west, though, has a reality of its own. The myths and legends were created, but the reality doesn't always fit the myth or legend — or even the general concept of what the west may be like. The modern west is changing as man seeks to use and/or change the environment.

The physical aspects of our environment are a large part of an individual's experience. They have an impact on the individual and the amount of stress and anxiety experienced. One aspect of the physical environment, i.e. population density, appears to have negative effects on feelings of personal security and on affiliative and other social responses to individuals or groups.

There has been relatively little research on crowding which has focused on individual and cross-cultural differences. Evans (1978) found evidence that young children may be more adversely affected by crowding than older persons. However, this may only be indicative of western cultures. Children in Kung society (Draper, 1974) apparently do not suffer any ill effects from crowding. Studies of crowding in Chicago (Galle, Gove, and MacPherson, 1972) support the hypothesis that pathology tends to increase as the population density increases. This relationship appears to work the other way in the Netherlands (Levy and Herzog, 1974). In a study done in Hong Kong, no adverse effects were found as the result of high population density (Mitchell, 1971).

The environment is the source of many stressors which can initiate a variety of reactions. These reactions may range from endocrine secretions to such things as complicated appraisals and evaluations of the sources. These reactions to stressors may be physiological (Selye, 1956) and/or psychological (Lazarus, Opton, & Tomita, 1966). Few investigators have attempted to study all aspects of the stress process simultaneously.

Stressful responses can be evoked by the changes and challenges that one experiences in daily life. They can be caused by the disruption of one's habits (e.g. unpredictable noise or crowding). Malfunctioning of social systems which place obstacles in one's path — deprivation, losses, and culturally-governed mores — may also contribute to stressful responses. Stressors may be intrusive, physical, and universally threatening (e.g. natural disasters). Others may be more culturally determined, less universal, and more psychosocial in nature. Aiello and Thompson (1980) found that varying intensities of crowding and proximities in spatial invasion are specific to cultural norms and meanings.

The obvious lack of relative crowding and the presence of generous open space in western rural areas would seem to offer escape from the stressors generally associated with urban areas. The lessening of noise factors, crowding, and other variables associated with stress production would seem to enhance the quality of life. In fact, these have been some of the traditional reasons why people have sought out rural areas for rest, relaxation, and vacations.

Ranchers and farmers have tended to form small close communities which have supported their way of life and provided for mutual support. Depending on their cultural heritage, they have developed and maintained values and attitudes congruent with their way of life. Other groups (e.g. Mexican Americans) have been generally successful in preserving their cultural heritages while attempting to adapt and adjust to changes in the United States' society. Others (e.g. Native American groups) have maintained their culture in varying degrees and, in many cases, in relative isolation from the mainstream of the U.S. society.

Much of the history of the United States is concerned with the westward expansion of a civilization that had its beginnings on the eastern shores of the North American continent. The Spaniards were the first men of European origins to penetrate the vast regions between the Rocky Mountains and the Pacific Ocean. As late as the 1820s, very little exploring had been done in the far west. In many cases, the terrain was found to be rough and rugged, and resources were scarce in the beginning. Communities were separated by great distances and travel was difficult, at best, by today's standards (Hulse, 1990).

Today, in many areas of the western United States, rural towns and communities may be separated by as much as 100 miles or more. Many of these towns are farm and ranch centers or mining towns. There is often a shortage of physicians, psychiatrists, and psychologists, as well as other mental health related services and trained personnel. An increase in population in a number of areas within the past 15–20 years has placed a tremendous strain on many local resources. The need for effective community counseling programs in rural areas of the western United States has been increasing. This is, at least partially, due to stressors placed on old timers and newcomers alike. The rapid growth in some areas is exacerbated by rapidly fluctuating economic changes. As more people enter an area, they tend to overwhelm old timers who, quite often, are left bewildered and lost in a community which once was theirs. Newcomers have difficulties dealing with scarce or non-existent services and resources as well as a lack of adequate housing. Tensions develop over these areas as well as from a clash of values. There is a need for adequate and effective community counseling centers to address these problem areas.

Human services in any community cover a broad area. In addition to mental health services, such services may include law enforcement, legal services, social services, public health, recreation, youth services, local government, educational services, and services for senior citizens. These services have generally been provided informally or through institutions. When rapid community growth occurs, the size of the local population may increase at a rate which causes people's problems to increase tremendously with a resultant strain on existing community resources.

In areas of rapid development, there tends to be a rapidly developing shortage of adequate and reasonably-priced housing. Rentals become high and crowding develops (Uhlmann, Doherty, and Hill, 1977). Recreation presents other problems. Citizens of rural communities in the west have traditionally engaged in recreational activities such as camping, fishing, and hunting. Newcomers tend to have a different set of interests (e.g. bowling alleys, theaters, swimming pools, and handball courts). Communities which can't provide these types of activities may find newcomers taking advantage of more easily available diversions such as drinking, gambling, and prostitution (Uhlmann, 1977).

Uhlmann (1977) pointed out a number of significant problem areas in her analysis of the delivery of human services in Wyoming boom towns. A review of her report points out the potential sources of stress and other mental health related problems encountered in western rural communities experiencing rapid growth. She found that mental health problems in rapidly developing communities include an increased incidence of depression among women and a rising rate of alcoholism among males. She also found an increase in family crises and that children and adolescents are at risk for an increased incidence of behavior disorders and social maladjustments. Newly arrived young adults (18–26) were found to face problems as a result of few, if any, solid interpersonal relationships. They frequently became involved in drug and alcohol abuse. Uhlmann found that public assistance through social services was drastically reduced and that there was frequently a lack of adequate medical personnel. She found that schools experienced difficulties as a result of a rapid growth in student population. At the high school level, the drop-out rate tended to increase as young people were attracted and drawn off by employment opportunities in the area.

Uhlmann suggested that law enforcement personnel in rapidly developing communities may have to deal with problems they have not encountered before and may be hampered by inadequate training, low salaries, and a high turnover of personnel. Poor and/or inadequate facilities (e.g. jails, juvenile detention, and foster homes) were seen as making the job of law enforcement more difficult.

Uhlmann has also suggested that local governments in small rural communities may not have the administrative structure necessary to deal with the new and critical demands placed on them by a rapidly growing population.

In the past, rural communities in the western United States were frequently characterized by a large population of senior citizens. Uhlmann suggests this occurred because young people left the community to seek better employment elsewhere. However, it seems that when a rapid increase in population due to development occurs, this process is partially reversed. Senior citizens may be forced to leave the community due to a rising cost of living. Such a process of demographic change was observed in three Wyoming communities (Uhlmann, Kimble, and Throgmorton, 1976; Uhlmann, Doherty, and Hill, 1977).

Other problems associated with rapid population growth include a sense of a decreasing "quality of life". Rapid growth brings rapid change. Many impacted communities have stressed decline and loss. The negative effects such accounts point out usually include: a speeded-up pace of life, congestion and overcrowding, inflation in prices, fear of change in life style for present residents, lack of activities and sense of belonging for newcomer families, alcoholism and mental health problems (*HUD Program Guide*, 1976). Increased incidents of severe depressions and alienation of both old-timers and newcomers may result in "we-they" conflicts.

Traditional agencies and persons who have dealt with the above problem areas may not even exist in such communities. Many of these small rural communities have long been used to everyone taking care of themselves. Existing agencies may find their caseloads overwhelming. Communities which are impacted need help in defining future problems, predicting the magnitude of such problems, and designing and implementing programs and mechanisms to alleviate the problems.

Uhlmann (1977) suggested that most of these problems develop because communities don't have the time to develop financial resource bases and local attitudinal support for needed services. She also suggested that problems occur due to the changing composition of local populations. She pointed out that all of the factors reviewed above bring about increased demands for human services in impacted communities.

Stress and Rural Areas

Stress in rural areas is often overlooked due to smaller populations. For example, Nevada has a history of boom and bust dating back to the middle of the nineteenth century (Hulse, 1990). As a state, it has managed to grow and expand its interests. Although geographically rugged and sparsely populated, it has maintained a rich culture and a pluralistic society. Basque sheepherders in the north, cattle ranchers, miners, Mexican Americans, Chinese Americans, Japanese Americans, Shoshone, Washo, and Paiute Indians, and many other groups add to the color and richness of Nevada culture.

Over the years, an expanded effort has been made to develop and maintain mental health services in rural areas (Doherty, 1984). Fluctuations in the economy have stressful effects on the small rural communities. Growth and decline of communities have a psychological impact on those directly affected. People experience this stress and anxiety differently, depending on a number of factors.

One method of studying perceived stress and anxiety is to use a self-report indicator such as Spielberger's (1970) State-Trait Anxiety Inventory (STAI). Spielberger (1970) states that Trait anxiety tends to be relatively stable and indicates a tendency to respond to situations perceived as threatening with elevations on the State scale. McClelland & Atkinson (2000) suggest that trait anxiety has the characteristics of a class of constructs which they term "motives". They define these as dispositions which remain latent until they are activated by cues in different situations. Campbell (See Spielberger & Bale, 1970) calls these "acquired behavioral dispositions". According to him, they involve residues of past experiences which tend to predispose individuals to view the world in a particular way. They also tend to predispose an individual to manifest what he calls "object consistent" response tendencies.

In other words, trait anxiety is like potential energy. It suggests differences between people in the disposition to respond to stressful situations with varying amounts of state anxiety (Spielberger & Bale, 1970). Persons with high levels of trait anxiety tend to be more likely to respond with an increase in state anxiety intensity in situations that hold a threat to their self-esteem (Spielberger & Bale, 1970). Whether persons who differ in trait anxiety differ in a similar way for state anxiety depends on the extent to which they perceive a specific situation as threatening or dangerous. This is strongly influenced by their past experiences.

Attitudes toward the sources of stress tend to mediate the responses. If an individual or a group believes that a stressor will cause no permanent harm, the response will probably be less extreme than if the danger poses the threat of lasting harm. Psychologically, the perceptions of control, social support, and other characteristics of individuals exposed to stressors will affect their evaluation of different stressors. Perceived control can be a powerful mediator of stress. That is, it can provide the individual, or group, with a sense of being able to cope more effectively.

Adequate needs assessments, community planning, and allocation of available human resources can help prevent and alleviate potential problems and stressors associated with rapidly growing rural communities. Such activities can give communities perceived and actual control over their futures and can contribute to the well-being and mental health of the whole community.

Changing Roles

In a longitudinal study, using preferences for living near family and in the local community obtained in the 8th and 11th grades, Elder, King, & Conger (1996) modeled the social and developmental pathways by which adolescents approach decisions to leave home and settle in other parts of the country. Data come from 351 two-parent families in the Iowa Youth and Family Project, launched in 1989 to investigate the economic stresses and family consequences of the farm crisis. Lack of socioeconomic opportunity; relatively weak and declining ties to parents, kin, and the religious community, and strong educational prospects emerged as strong sources of a declining preference for living near family and in the local community among boys and girls. Whether coupled with family attachments or not, plans to settle elsewhere after education were linked to more elevated feelings of depression and unhappiness about life.

Conger, Elder, & Lorenz (1994) examined the plight of several hundred rural families who lived through the years of economic hardship in the mid-1980s. The participants in the Iowa Youth and Families Project included farmers, people from small towns, and those who lost farms and other businesses as a result of the "farm crisis." Conger et al traced the influence of economic hardship on the emotions, behavior, and relationships of parents, children, siblings, husbands, and wives. They interviewed four members in each of 451 rural families. All of the families in the study included a seventh-grade adolescent, when they were interviewed in 1989. In addition to this target adolescent, both parents of the seventh-grader and a sibling within four years of age participated in the study. They were particularly concerned with the quality of social relationships, both within and outside the family, that might affect the various linkages in their theoretical model of family economic stress.

Cook & Heppner (1997) investigated the role of coping strategies, perceived control, and problem-solving appraisal in farmers' career transition processes. The sample, examined previously by P. P. Heppner et al (1991), included 79 male and female farmers (aged 39.2 and 41.6, respectively) who were participating in career transition workshops. Relationships among the three variables and an outcome variable, depressive symptomatology, were examined. Significant correlations were found between problem-solving appraisal and all other variables in this study.

Coping strategies were found to be related to depressive symptomatology. In a regression equation, only coping strategies contributed significantly, and no significant interaction was found between coping strategies and perceived control as hypothesized.

McInnes (2000) focused on the complex dynamics related to the family farm and their effect on the rural couple's relationship. The typical relationship examined was where the man is from a farming background and the woman from the city, or, if originally from the land, has lived or studied away from the district and been independent. The challenge for the counselor is to work with the two levels the couple bring:

- The couple's 'individual' story
- The larger context, including the man's family of origin, the family farm, the rural community, and the rural crisis nationally.

A case study of the typical couple's process and outcome in counseling was provided. It was concluded that the traditional stories about men, women, and relationships that once ordered the lives of couples on the land are no longer valid in times of enormous social and political change.

In life course theory, the principle of human agency states that "individuals construct their own life course through the choices and actions they take within the constraints and opportunities of history and social circumstances." Elder & Russell (2000) explore the implications of this principle, drawing upon three other principles of life course study:

- The location of individual lives in historical time and place.
- The differential timing of lives through events and experiences.
- Linked lives.

They focus on two historical periods in which adolescence was shaped by the agency of young people and their opportunities and constraints: the Great Depression of the 1930s, and the Great Farm Crisis and rural decline of the 1980s and 1990s. The resulting portrait is documented by research on lives in changing times over three decades. Within these historical eras, Elder & Russell view the agency of youth in terms defined by specific historical times and places. World War II played a major role in structuring pathways out of Depression disadvantage. Fifty years later, migration to urban areas of economic prosperity provided a general escape route for youth in the disadvantaged rural Midwest of the US. In each era, societal changes left their mark on the expression of human agency in youth's "negotiation of adolescence".

Conger, Rueter, & Conger (2000) present research from the Iowa Youth and Families Project (IYFP), a longitudinal study of Iowa families who were living in small towns and on farms during the farm crisis of the 1980s. The research was designed to assess how the macrosocial change and economic upheaval that occurred across the US during the 1980s influenced family functioning and the well-being of parents and their children. It describes the empirical and theoretical foundations for the Family Stress Model. The sections that follow summarize findings from the IYFP and other studies relevant to the various processes and mechanisms proposed in the Family Stress Model. They also consider research on hypothesized protective mechanisms or dimensions of vulnerability that may moderate the causal linkages proposed in the theoretical model. After reviewing the possible applied significance of this work, they close with a discussion of conclusions that can be drawn from the research conducted thus far and the implications of these findings for future investigations of family economic stress.

In another example, the crisis in the farming industry in the Netherlands has had far-reaching negative consequences for the well-being of farm-families. Based on identity-theory, Gorgievski-Duijvesteijn (1999) hypothesized that job-involvement (the psychological importance of the professional role) would intensify the negative relationship between role-relevant stressors and well-being. Specifically, 107 Dutch, self-employed dairy farm-couples (mean age 52 yrs for husbands and 49 yrs for wives) participated in a study that examined whether job-involvement exacerbates the negative effects of three role-relevant stressors (potential threats to business continuity, restrictions on autonomy as a self-employed person, and financial problems) on two indicators of well-being (job-related worrying and mental health complaints). Gender differences were also explored. Results show partial support for the hypotheses derived from identity-theory in that job-involvement only exacerbates the positive relationship between financial problems and job-related worrying for both spouses. No other moderating effects of job-involvement were found. Although husbands were more involved in farming than wives, the direct effect of the three role-relevant stressors on the two indicators of well-being were similar for both spouses.

During economic downturns, traditional gender allocations of labor have been considered to vary more than in prosperous times. While most studies have examined the division of labor in the household or in paid employment, Lobao &

Meyer (1995) examined it where both intersect, in family-owned and family-operated enterprises in the farm sector of the 1980s. This context, combining crisis conditions and the agency of economic actors, should be related to greater flexibility in labor allocations, leading to the feminization of farming. However, a contrasting perspective argues for rigidity of gender roles in farming. Lobao & Meyer use data from a twelve-state midwestern sample and a more detailed Ohio study. The results failed to support the flexibility thesis. The rigidity of production roles was further translated into different factors related to women's and men's stress.

DeFrain & Schroff (1991) examined how city life and country life differences influence parents in their efforts to rear children as well as endeavor to paint a more realistic picture of rural life. They begin with a section on the impact of urbanization on fathers and mothers in the United States, discussing the pluralistic nature of the city, the increased leisure of urban youth as compared to rural youth, the power of the youth peer group in urban areas, the impersonality and anonymity of the city, the pervasive nature of the urban mass media, and the urban ghetto. They focus on the positive aspects of urbanization: the advantages urban organization offers families and the relative affluence of the city compared to the country. They discuss special problems of rural fathers and mothers in the United States, including the dramatic decline in the farm population, the most recent wave of the continuing farm crisis, agricultural fundamentalism, resettlement, the impact of urbanization on farm parents and their children, the fact that the farm parents often find themselves preparing their children for an urban-industrial world that they themselves do not fully understand, the difficult realities of the rural economy today, and rural social class barriers farm families face.

Willson (1928) deals with the education of farm children and the relation of education to the migration of farmers to non-farming occupations. It is based upon original research of the author for Western North Dakota (N. Dak. Agr. Exper. Sta. Bull. 214, 1928) during the agricultural depression of 1920–1926. The data show that improved agricultural conditions and better financial returns from farming result in improved educational facilities and increased grade and high school attendance by farm children. A decrease in the number of farms did not operate to deprive the children of grade school education. The amount of high school education is decreased as distance from secondary schools and the proportion of foreign-born—especially the Russians—within the community are increased. The percentage of farm children in high schools is increasing. The percentage of farm children entering non-farming occupations increased directly with the amount of education they received. A point demonstrated in this study is the relationship between the ability to survive the agricultural crisis and type of family organization. The married individuals, who had children, survived the depression best of all.

Some Different Approaches

Peeks (1989) posits that school counselors must be ready to work with children of farm families in crisis to direct solutions to the presenting problems and provide the family with hope for the future. She notes that the problem of the student from a farm family can be viewed as a metaphor (mirroring the parents' own fears about the future and feelings of hopelessness) and a form of protection (diverting parental attention toward a solvable problem).

Mermelstein & Sundet (1998) focused on the decision criteria that influenced 118 directors of rural community mental health centers (CMHCs) as to whether to adopt innovative programming with regard to the crisis among farmers. Five criteria were postulated as independent variables:

- Compatibility with the director's values
- Relative advantage
- Observability
- Feasibility
- Trial-ability of the innovation

The dependent variables were the amount and type of farm crisis programming and the date of introduction into the Community Mental Health Center (CMHC). Findings demonstrate the widespread failure of CMHCs to respond effectively to mental health concerns arising from massive environmental stress. Impediments to innovation appear to be a real or perceived paucity of resources and a mentality favoring existing programs.

Peeks (1989) reviewed the transitions faced by adults from farm families whose farms have failed in the agriculture crisis, including career transition, relocating, a redefined lifestyle, and refocusing on future goals. Students' school problems are discussed as behavioral metaphors for the family's crisis, and a school-based strategy for counselors to help students, whose problems are related to the family transitions, is described. Six strategic interventions are presented for solving student problems by inviting the parents to school and focusing on positive problem-solving.

Paulsen (1988) asserts that the rural crisis is creating new numbers of rural individuals who are in need of assistance as they cope with the stress of economic dislocation and the overwhelming difficulties that occur after the loss of a farm or business. Individual, family, and community treatment aspects are discussed within the thematic context of a culture in crisis. An urban-based regional family service agency, Farmers Helping Farmers, is presented as an example of a system's response to the rural crisis. The proposed treatment involves a multilevel community response that includes self-help support groups, instruction of adaptive coping skills, and sharing information in rural communities. Mental health professionals are challenged to further their understanding of the rural crisis and to adopt more flexible treatment strategies to encompass a multilevel system's response.

Jurich & Russell (1987) evaluated 15 farm families, who underwent therapy at the Kansas State University Family Center, using a model of family adaptation to stress by H. I. McCubbin et al (see record 1981-30250-001). Major interventions included reframing, mobilizing resources, and utilizing less indirect means of intervention. Ss showed a greater increase in well-being at three months than did a general sample of clients. However, stress levels were not lowered as much as the general sample and life satisfaction was lower at follow-up than the general population.

Davis-Brown & Salamon (1987) argue that families' responses to the loss of their farm due to the agricultural crisis depend on whether shared agricultural goals originate primarily from financial or familial motivations. Salamon's (1985) farm management style types are combined with a family stress model by McCubbin and Patterson (1983) to develop a framework for identifying contrasting capabilities and definitions possessed by families holding divergent agricultural goals. An instrument based on the application of stress concepts to farm family research is presented for use in counseling families who lose their farms.

Rosenblatt (1990) offers testimony from 42 adults in 24 Minnesota farm couples that were caught in the farm crisis. They speak of how they struggled economically, what they understood and felt about their economic situation, and how their relationships within the family and outside of it were affected by the economic difficulties. The purpose was to go beneath the statistics, to record people's experiences, feelings, and reflections in their own words, and to understand what happened to them as individuals and families. That understanding has implications for policy, service delivery, and community action. Extensive face-to-face interviews were carried out in 1986 by three graduate students in the Department of Family

Social Science at the University of Minnesota. Telephone follow-up interviews were carried out in the latter half of 1987 and early part of 1988 with adults in 23 of the 24 households. Interviews were wide-ranging but focused mainly on the history of the farm operation, what happened in family and community relationships as economic difficulties developed, problems with lenders and creditors, and personal feelings and reflections as things happened. People were also asked to fill out a checklist of feelings, personal reactions, and aspects of family relationships that might be influenced by the crisis.

Ferguson & Engels (1989) discussed the 1980s farm crisis that had large numbers of farmers and their families abandoning farming due to new and frequently unmanageable economic realities. Selected issues were discussed with regard to farmers who:

- Were then working and living on family farms
- Were being or had been forced to pursue other occupations

Ferguson & Engels note that farmers are at a geographical disadvantage for receiving mental health and career counseling services, and most traditional support services are centered in keeping farmers in agriculture. Counselors and state and national counseling organizations need to consider pro bono and sponsored approaches for working with farm families. Farmers might benefit from modification of programs aimed at adult education, career development, retirement, and separation and grief.

Van Hook (1987) used the ABCX family-crisis model developed by Hill (1949) to identify needs and design intervention strategies while long-term solutions to the crisis are being developed. Basic to the model is the concept that each event has not only an external reality but an internally experienced reality as well. Van Hook suggested that focusing on the family unit strengthens both individual and family resources. Because many farm families have considerable strengths, relatively small intervention efforts may be needed to enable them to mobilize for survival.

Telecounseling

Counseling by telephone further lends itself well to disaster and traumatic response. Because victims may be overwhelmed by immediate on-site counselor response and may need time to grieve or otherwise react, providing the means to follow up by telephone at one's convenience as needed has strong appeal. A system of referral through such methods as distributing business-sized cards at the site with an 800 number to call when needed and in which the client initiates the process is both responsive and unobtrusive.

Despite all the challenges involved, a counselor-staffed telephone-response system to disaster and trauma offers supports long after the crisis. Such telecounseling offers them support immediately, when the victim is in crisis, conveniently, and anonymously. It cuts through distance, class, appearances, and resistances to therapy. It is a lifeline to engaging the victim at any point.

Telephone counseling additionally presents itself well to disaster and traumatic response since victims may initially be overwhelmed by their experiences and be resistant to using treatment; yet may later need to access counseling services. Through telephone contact, this can be done in a non-threatening way as their grieving and symptoms unfold. As a result, telephone counseling is both responsive to the victim and can be an effective point of access to the therapeutic process.

To summarize, it is important that the mental health profession be aware of the factors involved in rural crises—socially, economically, community-wide, and on other related variables. Providing appropriate responses, approaches, methods, and programs that are individualized for communities and individuals is important in these times of change and increased levels of stress.

Rural Trauma

Background and the Problems

Within one year, in the early 1990s, a small rural American town experienced a series of traumatic events. A number of individuals put in much time and effort toward a crisis plan, known as the *Trauma Intervention Plan*, which ultimately failed. Taplitz-Levy (2002) explored the factors that added to and detracted from the success of the specific school-based collaborative intervention and research project. The attitudes of crisis team members toward the crisis plans, collaborative work, and research were examined using a series of qualitative research methods. Through qualitative analysis of the data, results show that the Trauma Intervention Plan was hindered by poor communication, a lack of trust, and poor historical relationships between the school team and the out-of-school consultants. Taplitz-Levy's study gives compelling reasons for school personnel and local community mental health staff to develop positive relationships.

In June 1981, southeastern Kentucky experienced serious and widespread flooding. In May 1984, a storm system brought tornadoes, strong winds, and severe, extensive flooding to this same area. Norris, Phifer, & Kaniasty (1994) studied the psychosocial impact of these events. Their study had three features that hold particular promise for increasing what we know about the effects of disaster:

- The study's prospective and longitudinal design
- Its consideration of both individual and collective aspects of disaster exposure
- Its focus on older people (age 55 or older)

This study addressed the following questions:

- What impact did these two floods have upon the mental, physical, and social functioning of the rural Appalachian victims?
- Were these individuals able to take these events "in stride" or did they present a serious challenge to their ability to cope?
- Did these floods leave a lasting impact on the mental and physical well-being of these individuals or did they only result in relatively minor and short-lived emotional upset?
- Were some people more affected than others?
- Were these communities able to "rally around" their members or were they shattered and split apart?

In September 1991, in the small rural town of Hamlet, NC, a fryer exploded at a chicken processing plant, killing 25 employees and injuring many more. This disaster stirred national attention, influenced state law and inspection policies, and profoundly affected the entire community. Derosa (1995) examined the relationship between PTSD and the survivors' subjective experiences of the trauma, their search for meaning, and their perceptions of self, of others, and of the world around them. They attempted to capture the survivors' experiences of themes such as rage, grief, and a belief in a benevolent world, in conjunction with clinical diagnosis of PTSD (using the SCID interview) in order to assess the buffering or exacerbating influence of the subjective experience. Seventy-eight subjects included the plant's employees, relatives of employees, rescue personnel, and relatives of fire/rescue personnel. They examined several categories of variables:

- Unresolved trauma themes
- 'Pre-fire' variables including neuroticism
- History of traumatic experiences

- Previous psychiatric treatment
- "Peri-traumatic" variables including dissociation injury, and , fear of level of exposure to the fire
- Types of social support
- Demographics

The most robust variables contributing to lifetime diagnosis of PTSD after the fire were having lower socio-economic status, being female, feeling little social support, fearing death/injury, and dissociating during the fire. The only significant contribution to the model for chronic PTSD was the number of unresolved trauma themes. The degree to which the trauma themes remained maladaptive varied by the severity of diagnosis. Exploratory cluster analyses of patterns of unresolved themes among survivors and their families suggested that in addition to the number of unresolved themes, the pattern of thematic resolution is associated with diagnosis.

In 1992, El Salvador ended a twelve-year civil war which caused tremendous social upheaval. Approximately 50,000 civilians were killed, 500,000 displaced, and 750,000 to one million left the country (Lundgren and Lang, 1994). The impact of the violence left many survivors with traumatic emotional problems. Oakes (1998) studied three rural communities in El Salvador. She examined the emotional reactions of eighty respondents to war, analyzing the data from the point of view of respondents. Respondents included those who had only indirect war experiences, those who experienced occasional traumatic events during the war, and those who lived in a war zone and had continuous and extreme experiences during the war. Respondents reacted to everyday events, violence, and war with an escalating pattern of emotions. This pattern began with worries often connected to everyday events, then fears often related to violence, and then to emotional states including "ataques de nervios" and affliction, and finally to sadness caused by loss. Some physical reactions related specifically to war, such as jumping at noise; while others, such as headaches, were experienced by all, regardless of the amount or type of war experience. Past war experiences often affected how respondents reacted emotionally to everyday events in the present, especially when those events were linked to danger or violence. Respondents who had only indirect exposure to war reacted to present and future events only occasionally and mildly through the standpoint of past events in war, while individuals who had prolonged and extreme war experiences reacted to present and future events much more intensely and regularly through the viewpoint of war. In an additional analysis of a small group of respondents who had lived through extreme warfare, Oakes reported that they had few emotional reactions to normal events that they did not relate to war. She suggested that the sum of many people's emotional reactions, therefore, may cause such configurations of people to have reactions to events that are not based on present reality.

Since 1994, lethal violence toward people suspected of witchcraft has escalated in rural communities in South Africa. Hundreds of older people believed to be witches have been burned to death and thousands, who escaped death, have taken refuge in government established camps. Hill (2000) examined a group counseling approach that promotes "sustainable reconciliation" with traumatized individuals in communities divided by violence due to witchcraft persecution. Specifically, Hill examined a single case sample of a group counseling session aimed at reconciliation. Fifteen group members included individuals from conflictual parties from geographic areas in South Africa where there are witch burnings. Beyond the 15 group members, 11 other participants rated the group session and its potential for fostering sustainable reconciliation. These 11 individuals were divided into two groups:

- American student raters   (N = 3)
- South African observers   (N = 8).

This study was constructed as a 10-step process of data gathering and a "constant comparison" (Strauss & Corbin, 1994) of data categorized by all participants. As defined by Glaser and Strauss (1967), the Grounded Theory methodology allowed for an emergence of common themes across raters that could be related to theories for sustainable reconciliation, trauma counseling, group process, and witchcraft persecution. The results of this study suggest that sustainable peace is possible using the "reconciliation group counseling" approach. With these specific types of groups, special consideration must be given to leadership style, building safety, and including the entire community that has been affected by witch persecution. However, according to participants, reconciliation groups will fail if the fundamental reasons for the violence continue to go unattended (e.g., poverty, unemployment, etc). Such fundamental issues perpetuate feelings of fear and hopelessness in community members, which fosters an unstable environment. These results suggest that therapists must understand the context of such violence, attend to the trauma symptoms of individuals, and perhaps play a supportive role in the group. The South African observers suggested that successive counseling groups, with public admittance of behavior and retribution for losses, would be necessary before sustainable peace could be possible.

The above studies have identified variables, approaches, and interventions, and make suggestions for a variety of events that produced trauma in rural areas. The following section presents results of studies involving the effects of various trauma-producing events on children, parents, and families.

Baden (1998) discusses how newspapers seem to be telling us that every cornfield is threatened by a Dairy Queen restaurant. This media barrage about the crisis of our "shrinking" farmland is traced to the 1979 publication of "Where Have All the Farmlands Gone?" by the National Agricultural Lands (NALS) Study. The NALS report, to which eleven federal agencies contributed, argued that land-use planning and control must be employed to protect valuable farmland from "urban sprawl".

Baden's edited book, a collection of essays by a distinguished group of economists including Theodore W. Schulz, Julian L. Simon, and Pierre Crosson, takes issue with the belief that croplands need governmental protection. In opposition, the collection as a whole supports two theses:

- Shrinking farm acreage is not a serious problem

- Individual choices by landowners in a market setting result in better organized land use than would governmental land-use planning and regulation

Throughout, large parts of the developing world's rural livelihoods are in crisis (Bernstein, Crow, and Johnson, 1992). Even in those parts of the third world where there has been growth of food output, that growth has rarely been translated into a commensurate expansion of livelihoods. Bernstein et al (1992) examined how people in developing countries survive and how their lives have been affected by the great changes since the World War II. They examined the diverse human implications of rural change, the various crises of rural livelihoods which arise from change, and the survival strategies of individuals and households. They describe the great processes of agrarian transformation which have fundamentally altered rural livelihoods in developing countries, identifying some of the dilemmas for public action which arise from agrarian transformation and the crises of rural livelihoods. The contributors draw on a range of disciplinary approaches to the subject— including anthropology, sociology, economics, political economy, agricultural science, and development studies.

Not only does the culture of rurality have differences from urban areas, but rural cross-cultural differences are also important in understanding and providing appropriate responses and services to residents of rural environments. Further attention and study of these areas as well as the awareness of what is already known is needed to inform mental health and other professionals working in these areas.

Domestic Violence

Domestic violence and poverty are interwoven. Poverty makes it difficult to deal with domestic violence and undermines financial stability and possible strategies for effective change. Significant numbers of low-income women in the rural western US are battered, and the violence they experience can make their climb out of poverty impossible. Poverty, in turn, makes it more difficult to end domestic violence and heal its effects. Without long-term financial stability, reducing the risk of physical violence does not make battered women and their children safe. While focusing on physically separating the battered woman and her children from the abusive partner, most criminal justice interventions overlook basic needs: a roof over their heads, food on their table, or available health care.

Partner violence is a serious mental and physical health concern leading to debilitating physical injury in women. Significant psychological sequelae are associated with battering. However, only recent investigations have begun to delineate the different types of psychological distress. The diagnosis of Post-traumatic Stress Disorder (PTSD) has been useful in characterizing the symptoms associated with victims of severe trauma. The DSM-IV criteria for PTSD include re-experiencing trauma, avoidance responses, and heightened arousal. Given the characteristics shared between battered women and other victims of violent crime, Presty (1996) predicted that battered women develop primary features of PTSD. The second hypothesis was that other women would meet DSM-IV criteria for Acute Stress Disorder (ASD). She also performed exploratory analyses to examine relationships between the frequency and severity of abuse and diagnostic categories. The results confirmed the two hypotheses. First, 65.6% of the sample was PTSD positive, with 5% meeting criteria for ASD. Other anxiety disorders accounted for 13.1%. The prevalence rate of Major Depressive Disorder (MDD) was 70.5%. The comorbidity of depression with PTSD was 84.6%. Physical abuse significantly predicted PTSD development, explaining 11.4% of the total variance. Verbal abuse significantly predicted MDD. Dissociation was predicted by both verbal and physical abuse. Exploratory cluster analysis revealed three typologies of battered women:

- Cluster 1 reflected young, poorly educated women, who experienced the greatest physical and sexual abuse. They had the highest levels of PTSD, moderate depression, and the poorest level of functioning.

- Cluster 2 women were the oldest, had the most children, and had the longest relationship duration. They experienced more verbal than physical abuse, and had the highest degree of depression, with modest PTSD severity.

- Cluster 3 reflected the youngest, most educated group, with the least number of children, and shortest relationship duration.

Wendt, Taylor, & Kennedy (2002) provide a critique of the Australian research into rural domestic violence. Research to date has focused on the factors that keep rural women trapped in violent relationships. While this research has been useful in developing policy to address rural domestic violence, it has not yet provided information about women's understandings of their rural contexts. Research into domestic violence is moving toward acknowledging and recognizing the complexities and differences between people's experiences. Wendt et al suggest that it is time to explore the differences between various rural regions and to move away from the assumption that there is one rural culture. They suggest that a move towards feminist post-structural perspectives has strengths in that it enables a focus on the meanings of rural cultures from the perspectives of women, who experience, and men, who perpetrate domestic violence. If these meanings become apparent, it may enable local solutions to be implemented and contribute knowledge and new ideas.

Although it has been suggested frequently that certain aspects of rural culture present barriers to women escaping domestic violence, research has not yet focused on how rural culture affects women's experiences. Wendt & Cheers (2002) report a study that explored how 14 rural women experiencing domestic violence perceived local cultural beliefs and values, the extent to which they had internalized these, and how they believed rural culture affected them in their situations. Components of their local rural cultures that they identified as impacting on their experiences of domestic violence included: belief in the sanctity and permanence of marriage, the importance and privacy of the nuclear family, Christian doctrine, and preservation of intergenerational property transfer. Each woman's story shows that, while rural culture gave them strength to endure the violence, it also created internal conflicts between wanting to escape and the cultural beliefs and values that they had internalized. Also, they were afraid of community reactions in case they left. Consequently, they did not disclose their violent situation and persevered in them far longer than they thought they would have in a different cultural context.

Youth Violence

Slovak (2000, 2001, 2002) addressed gaps in the youth violence literature by exploring the types and levels of children's exposure to violence in a rural setting. She also examined the psychological trauma associated with exposure to violence. Her initial study (Slovak, 2000) was a secondary data analysis which utilized the rural sample (N=549) from a larger study. The larger study had conducted a 45 minute questionnaire with students in grades 3 through 8. The questionnaire was designed to tap into children's present and past exposure to violence as a victim and witness across the home, school, and neighborhood. This questionnaire also assessed children's trauma symptoms.

Slovak found that children in the rural sample were exposed to high amounts of violence as both a victim and witness within and prior to the past year. In general, more boys reported being victims or witnesses to an at-least-sometimes violent event within the past year compared to girls, except for the act of being touched in a private place. In addition, more students in the lower grades reported being the victims and witnesses of violent acts compared to students in upper grades. Students reported that home was the place where they were most likely to be victims of violence, with the school being the next most likely place to be victimized, at least sometimes. The neighborhood was reported as the least likely place for students to be victims of violence, at least sometimes within the past year. Students reported a different trend for witnessing violence. They reported that school was the most likely place to witness violence, with the neighborhood being second. The home was the site reported as the least likely place to witness violence, at least sometimes within the past year. Slovak also found that exposure to violence variables explained a significant amount of variance in anxiety, anger, dissociation, depression, PTSD, and total trauma score above demographic variables. This is consistent with the literature examining the association of trauma and exposure to violence. These findings can be utilized to inform policy, practice, and research conducted in rural areas. In addition, the documentation of children's exposure to violence in a rural setting can help banish the stereotype that rural communities are safe havens from violence.

Peltzer (1999) identified exposure to experiences such as violence and the consequences for health in children in a rural South African community. The stratified random sample included 68 (46%) boys and 80 (54%) girls in the age range of 6–16 years. Their ethnicity was Northern Sotho. The interviews included the Children's Posttraumatic Stress Disorder Inventory and the Reporting Questionnaire for Children. They grouped experiences into either traumatic or other events. 99 (67%) had directly or vicariously experienced a traumatic event which included witnessing someone killed or seriously injured, a serious accident, a violent or very unexpected death or suicide of a loved one, sexual abuse or rape of a relative or friend, violent crime, child abuse, and other life-threatening situations. Scores on the Children's Posttraumatic Stress Disorder Inventory of 17 (8.4%) fulfilled the criterion for posttraumatic stress disorder (PTSD). 71% had more than one score and 53% had more than four scores on the Reporting Questionnaire for Children. Posttraumatic stress symptoms were significantly related to age and experiences such as those mentioned above.

Gun Violence

Slovak and Singer (2001) compared rural youth (Grades 3-8) exposed to gun violence and rural youth not exposed to gun violence on a number of variables: anger, anxiety, dissociation, depression, posttraumatic stress, total trauma, violent behavior, parental monitoring, and levels of violence in the home, school, and community. One-fourth (25%) of the 549 subjects reported having been exposed to gun violence at least once. Youth exposed to gun violence reported significantly more anger, dissociation, posttraumatic stress, and total trauma. In addition, youth exposed to the violence of guns reported significantly higher levels of violent behaviors and exposure to violence in other settings and also reported lower levels of parental monitoring. This study contributed to the growing body of literature addressing the stereotype that rural communities are not immune to the violence of firearms. This stereotype can act as a barrier to mental health practice, research, and policy issues in rural communities.

Slovak (2002) investigated the relationship between access to firearms and parental monitoring on rural youths' exposure to gun violence and examined the effect of gun violence exposure on the mental health of these youths, She administered a survey to 162 students (mean age 14.3 years) who participated in a student assistance program that provided in-school support groups for students in grades 6 through 12. Her results show that a substantial number were exposed to gun violence and exposure was significantly related to firearm access and parental monitoring. Furthermore, gun violence exposure was significantly associated with trauma among the youths. Implications for mental health workers include advising high-risk clients and their families on gun removal and safe storage practices.

Suicide/Murder in Rural Areas

Suicide can occur as a response to increased perceived stress and can also be a response to a severe loss. Treatments for suicidal ideation in rural areas are very limited. Dimmick, Burgiss, & Robbins (2003) assessed the impact of a suicide intervention program from a consumer perspective. Self-administered question-naires were distributed to consumers who had been referred to a suicide interven-tion counselor in the two-year period of the program in rural southwest Western Australia. 35 patients completed and returned the questionnaire. Three-quarters of respondents were positive about their experience with the service, with half of the respondents no longer having thoughts of suicide and only 20% of all respondents reporting having attempted deliberate self-harm post-counseling. Reported suicidal ideation and attempted self-harm were much higher in the dissatisfied group. Dissatisfaction of respondents stemmed from the history of their treatment and "the hassle created by the many systems for them to access care". However, the overall outcome of this study is that, from the consumers' perspective, a high-intensity approach to suicide intervention resolved or improved the presenting problem and their ability to deal with it.

Ragland & Berman (1990-1991) examined the relationship between the farm economic crisis and farmer suicide rates, using data from 15 states in the US from 1980 to 1985. Suicide frequencies for farmers and two control occupations (forestry and transportation workers) were obtained. The 1980 US Census occupational population data were used to convert these frequencies into suicide rates. Suicide rates for farmers were greater than rates for transportation workers (truck drivers), but no different from rates for forestry workers. A significant positive correlation between the declining farm economy and increasing state suicide rates was also found.

2 Culture and Rurality

Culture refers to the shared attributes—including beliefs, norms, and values—of a group of people (DHHS, 2001). Peoples' reactions to disaster and their coping skills, as well as their receptivity to crisis counseling, differ significantly because of their individual beliefs, cultural traditions, and economic and social status in the community. For this reason, workers in our nation's public health and human services systems increasingly recognize the importance of cultural competence in the development, planning, and delivery of effective disaster mental health services.

Cultural Competence

There are many terms used in referring to concepts that are associated with cultural competence. They are used also in reference to interactions between and among people of different cultures. Such terms include *cultural diversity, cultural awareness, cultural sensitivity, multiculturalism, and transcultural services,* etc. The differences in the meanings of these terms may be subtle. However, they are extremely important. For example, the term *cultural awareness* suggests that it may be sufficient for one to be cognizant, observant, and conscious of similarities and differences among cultural groups (Goode et al., 2001). *Cultural sensitivity,* on the other hand, suggests the ability to empathize with and understand the needs and emotions of persons of one's own culture as well as those of others and to identify with emotional expressions and the problems, struggles, and joys of someone from another culture (Hernandez and Isaacs, 1998).

The term *cultural competence* suggests a broader concept than *cultural sensitivity*. The word *competence* implies the capacity to function effectively, both at the individual and organizational levels. *Competence* is associated with *culture* in order to emphasize that being aware of or sensitive to the differences between cultures is not sufficient. Instead, service providers must have the knowledge, skills, attitudes, policies, and structures needed to offer support and care that is responsive and tailored to the needs of culturally diverse population groups. Many people and organizations have developed definitions of cultural competence. The following definition blends elements of definitions used by SAMSHA (DHHS, 2001), the Health Resources and Services Administration (DHHS), the Office of Minority Health (DHHS, 2000a), and definitions found in the literature (Bazron and Scallet, 1998; Cross et al., 1989; Denboba, 1993; Evans, 1995; Roberts et al.,1990; Taylor et al., 1998):

> Cultural competence is a set of values, behaviors, attitudes, and practices within a system, organization, program, or among individuals that enables people to work effectively across cultures. It refers to the ability to honor and respect the beliefs, language, interpersonal styles, and behaviors of individuals and families receiving services, as well as staff who are providing such services. Cultural competence is a dynamic, ongoing, developmental process that requires a long-term commitment and is achieved over time.

Cross et al. (1989) note that culturally competent organizations and individuals:

- Value diversity
- Have the capacity for cultural assessment
- Are aware of cross-cultural dynamics
- Develop cultural knowledge
- Adapt service delivery to reflect an understanding of cultural diversity

At the individual level, cultural competence requires an understanding of one's own culture and worldview as well as those of others. It involves an examination of one's attitudes, values, and beliefs, and the ability to demonstrate values, knowledge, skills, and attributes needed to work sensitively and effectively in cross-cultural situations (Goode et al., 2001).

At the organizational and programmatic levels, cultural competence requires a comprehensive, coordinated plan that cuts across policymaking, infrastructure building, program administration and evaluation, and service delivery. Culturally competent organizations and programs acknowledge and incorporate the importance of culture, assess cross-cultural relations, are aware of dynamics that can result from cultural differences and ethnocentric attitudes, expand cultural knowledge, and adopt services that meet unique cultural needs (DHHS, 2000d).

Cultural competence is not a matter of being politically correct or of assigning one person to handle diversity issues. It does not mean simply translating materials into other languages. Instead, it is an ongoing process of organizational and individual development which includes learning more about our own and other cultures. It alters our thinking about culture, based on what we learn, and changes the ways in which we interact with others. It reflects an awareness and sensitivity to diverse cultures. The *Cultural Competence Continuum* was developed by Cross et al. (1989) for mental health professionals. Today, many other public health practitioners and community-based service providers also find it as a useful tool. The continuum assumes that cultural competence is a dynamic process with multiple levels of achievement. It can be used to assess an organization's or individual's level of cultural competence, to establish benchmarks, and to measure progress.

The negative end of the continuum is characterized by *cultural destructiveness*. Organizations or individuals in this stage view cultural differences as a problem and participate in activities that purposely attempt to destroy a culture. Examples of destructive actions include denying people of color access to their natural helpers or healers, removing children of color from their families on the basis of race, and risking the wellbeing of minority individuals by involving them in social or medical experiments without their knowledge or consent. Organizations and individuals at this extreme operate on the assumption that one race is superior and that it should eradicate "lesser" cultures.

Special Populations in Rural Areas

Rural Families and Children

Rural families and children in rural areas encounter situations different from their urban counterparts. Cowen (2001) described the sociodemographic and stress characteristics of rural parents who accessed crisis child care services and determined if the utilization of these services would reduce the reported incidence of child maltreatment. 127 sets of parents (aged 17–62) completed a basic sociodemograpbic questionnaire and the Parenting Stress Inventory (PSI). Child maltreatment reporting statistics were used to determine if there was a significant decrease in the reported incidence of child maltreatment. The demographic data suggested economic disadvantage. The data indicated that parents perceived external stressors, those outside of the parent-child relationship, as the major contributor to their current life crisis. Comparison of child maltreatment rates between rural communities that did and did not receive crisis child care preventive interventions indicated that the programs were effective in preventing child maltreatment. The findings of this study provide support for the ecological model of child maltreatment which posits that availability of social support for families that experience high stress or crisis can decrease the incidence of child maltreatment.

Various types of crisis intervention are often used in rural environments. Anderson (1976) presents a variation of short-term family crisis treatment adapted to the specific needs of rural families in northern New Hampshire. Crisis was defined as a significant loss, and treatment consisted of 5–6 sessions which incorporated contract setting and homework assignments. She suggests that crisis intervention may be the treatment of choice in a rural setting.

The importance of families and the responses of children to disasters in rural areas have been studied by a number of groups following natural disasters. In February 1955, tornadoes destroyed two rural schoolhouses in Mississippi, both killing teachers and many of the students. A case study of a limited number of the families involved was initiated to investigate the processes by which a family, in the context of its community and subculture, may deal with the traumatic experiences of disaster. In certain areas, the data of this study can be compared with data of a previous study of children in disaster, i.e. "The Child and his Family in Disaster: A Study of the 1953 Vicksburg Tornado" (Perry & Perry, 1959).

Earls, Smith, & Reich (1988) report on a pilot study examining the reactions of children to a disaster of severe flooding in a circumscribed area of rural Missouri. Both parents and 6–17 yr old children (32 parent-child pairs) were interviewed separately, approximately one year after the flood, using parallel versions of a structured diagnostic interview designed to identify children with Diagnostic and Statistical Manual of Mental Disorders (DSM-III) diagnoses. Results document the importance of interviewing children directly. Children reported more anxiety symptoms than parents reported for their children. Although symptoms of posttraumatic stress were reported, none of the children met full criteria for the disorder. Children most likely to be adversely affected were those with a pre-existing disorder and those with parents who also reported a high number of symptoms in themselves.

In another study of post-disaster effects on children, 32 mothers and their children (aged 6–17 yrs) who had been exposed to severe flooding in rural Mississippi were interviewed, using the Diagnostic Interview for Children and Adolescents. Other sources of information about the children included school reports and the teachers' version of the Child Behavior Checklist. Results indicated that in most cases of psychiatric disorder, the diagnosis could have been made from the child's report alone. Children as young as six years of age reported emotional problems of which the parent appeared unaware. The decision-making process used in the assignment of summary psychiatric diagnoses based on child and parent reports as well as a number of other sources of information about the child are important factors to consider when doing assessments (Reich & Earls, 1987).

The farm crisis in the 1980s provided some insights into how rural families cope with crises. For example, data from 77 adolescents in farm and ranch families were used to examine the relationship of demographic variables, family stressor events, and family coping strategies to adolescent adaptation (Plunkett, Henry, & Knaub, 1999). Results indicated that adolescent age and family transitions were positively related to individual stress. Males reported less family stress than did females. Seeking spiritual support was negatively related to family stress while the perceived impact of the farm crisis was positively related to family stress. Family support was positively related, and family substance use issues were negatively related, to adolescent satisfaction with family life.

Forrest (1988) contends that the rural family, with its particular stressors, is increasingly vulnerable to overwhelming crises. She hypothesizes that adolescent suicide, although rare, may result from or add to that stress.

Thompson & McCubbin (1987) outline resource materials available to help educators, counselors, and others to support rural families in crises and facilitate decision making, long-range planning, and problem solving. Counseling programs, workshops, publications, support groups for coping with stress, and computerized decision aids are reviewed.

Children

Children are resilient and vulnerable at the same time. They are typically very healthy physically and even when injured, they recover quickly. They are often in the care of loving, supportive caregivers. Many social and educational resources exist to provide a positive and productive atmosphere of growth and development for children.

Rural children are often active in community activities, schools, churches, and clubs. Even with social support, rural children are at risk and should be targeted by the crisis counseling program. Disasters disrupt the daily lives of children and cause stress that can result in physical and emotional sequelae. According to *Taking Rural Into Account: Report on the National Public Forum* (CMHS, 1993), *a* disproportionate number of rural children are at high risk for mental disorders and live in poverty.

Several factors make outreach efforts to children a high priority:

- Children experience the same cognitive, physical, emotional, and spiritual reactions as adults. However, they lack experience in dealing with stress, vocabulary to express themselves, and conceptual ability to form a well-rounded perspective.

- Children have limited perspectives on life-events and are more dependent on others than adults.

- Children may have experienced the injury or death of a family member or friend in the disaster.

- There may have been significant damage or total loss of home or possessions.

- Children and their family may have moved due to the disaster.

- Parents may be unusually preoccupied with their own disaster response.

Children may lack verbal skills for expressing their concerns and thoughts. They have not developed the cognitive skills needed to interpret their experience. Children communicate through play, imaginative story, and art. Few adults take the time or have the insight to grasp the significance of such communication. Children are physically smaller than adults. This may not seem significant, but it does contribute to the ease with which they are often "lost in the shuffle" or "overlooked" by the adults around them. They may have to escalate attention-getting behaviors in the chaos of disaster recovery. They will express their hurt to adults who are hurting as well. Parental adjustment directly impacts the emotional recovery of children (CMHS, 1996).

The nature of rural family farm businesses is another factor to consider when targeting children for crisis counseling services. Children whose parents' family business is farming are often required by necessity to assume certain farm chores as a part of their typical family/household chores. After the disaster happens, there is often the expectation that they will assist their parents with farm-related disaster clean-up chores. Sometimes this may mean long absences from school or community activities.

Families, schools, churches, and other groups responsible for providing care and service to children may be the most likely sources of access to rural children affected by disaster. These resources are often difficult to collaborate with and may require some diplomacy or an "in" with the establishment. Balancing the need to provide services for children with the need to be respectful of the parents, teachers, and other caregivers is a challenge for almost every crisis counseling program.

A package of services designed to address and serve the needs of schools should be developed. Various schools in disaster affected areas have different levels of need for services and, at times, different perceptions of need. Because of this, marketing crisis counseling services to schools cannot be a "one size fits all" approach. Tailoring a package of services on an individual basis with each school is one way to enhance the potential for gaining access. School administrators and key staff need to understand that the Crisis Counseling Program exists to help them deal with these potentially disruptive and troubling issues in their school.

Whole school assemblies, small groups, one-on-one counseling, peer counseling, consultation, and training are effective approaches for reaching teachers and other staff. School-based activities that may be useful include: disaster-related coloring books, poster contests, poem writing, song writing, essay writing, art therapy, puppet programs, skits, and service projects.

If the disaster has impacted the local school(s), rural students may have to travel a great distance to a neighboring school or attend a makeshift school in a facility that is overcrowded. Some administrators are concerned that providing any program dealing with the disaster will only create more disturbance in the school. However, experience has shown that the opposite is more often the case. The anxiety and related energy levels of children in disaster affected areas often result in various levels of chaos if not given a productive outlet. Interactive programs, such as those mentioned above, provide a positive alternative to loss of interest in school work and acting out while promoting discussion and expression of feelings.

Elderly in Rural Areas

As America ages and the impending impact of the Baby Boom generation is only a few years away, it is important to look seriously at how rural elderly do in our society. Snustad, Thompson-Heisterman, & Neese (1993) explored the special challenges confronting a multi-disciplinary team attempting mental health outreach to rural elders. The services that are provided and the principles that guide these services are discussed and illustrated by case studies. Although the program is designed to be appropriate for epidemiology demography, topography, social and cultural environment, and economic and resource infrastructure of the rural southeast, these services and principles can be readily extended to other geographic areas.

Developing approaches that fit in rural communities and take into account the specific demographics of rural environments will continue to be critical in providing adequate care for rural elderly.

Snustad, Thompson-Heisterman, & Neese (1993) explored the special challenges confronting a multi-disciplinary team attempting mental health outreach to rural elders. Outreach services offer an approach to increasing the equity and accessibility of mental health services to this at-risk population. The services that are provided and the principles that guide these services are discussed and illustrated by case studies. Services include:

- Multidisciplinary assessment and intervention
- Integrating community services
- Assuming access
- Counseling
- Caregiver support
- Family counseling
- Psychiatric diagnosis and treatment
- Crisis intervention
- Advocacy

Although the program is designed to be appropriate for epidemiology demography, topography, social and cultural environment, and economic and resource infrastructure of the rural southeast, these services and principles can be readily extended to other geographic areas.

Hospitalization for various problems in rural areas can be problematic when large geographic areas are involved, when there is a lack of professionals in rural areas and when other resources including the close availability of hospitals is not existent. Neese, Abraham, & Buckwalter, (1999) developed predictive models of psychiatric hospitalization, use of mental health services, and use of crisis intervention by 152 rural elders (mean age 78 yrs) participating in an outreach case-management program. A combination of demographic, health status, and organizational variables were used in stepwise multiple regression. Ss completed the Mini-Mental Health State Examination and psychiatric diagnoses were classified according to Diagnostic and Statistical Manual of Mental Disorders-III-Revised (DSM-III-R). Being married and having supplemental insurance in addition to Medicare predicted 23% of the variance for utilization of psychiatric hospitalization. Only one variable, Medicaid, predicted 14% of the variance for use of mental health services. Type of caregiver, marital status, household composition, and Medicaid insurance accounted for 23% of the variance in utilization of crisis intervention by rural elders. Overall, the two variables that most likely predicted the use of psychiatric mental health services were marital status and type of insurance.

Developing approaches that fit in rural communities and take into account the specific demographics of rural environments will continue to be critical in providing adequate care for rural elderly.

Older Adults

It is important to note that older adults are concentrated in the central parts of metropolitan areas, but also heavily populate the small, rural towns across the country. Compared to their urban counterparts, rural older adults are in poorer health, have lower incomes, and are more restricted and isolated by inadequate transportation.

Becoming old means facing a time of transition and changing roles and is a stage of life that increases the likelihood of psychological problems such as low self-esteem and depression. Older adults have the highest suicide rate of any age group in American society. They also tend to be socially isolated. In rural areas, geographic isolation may compound social isolation. Adequate social support mitigates these problems.

This life phase also includes role shifts of retirement, widowhood, and death. Often, children move far away. Health problems develop that can lead to loss of mobility and independence. The older adult encounters many losses during this stage of life. A disaster only magnifies these issues, particularly if older adults have experienced loss of their home and material possessions including treasured mementos of a life time that cannot be replaced. Older rural adults who have lost not only their homes but farming businesses as well are particularly at high risk. The additional stressor associated with loss of income/livelihood is a special factor to consider when providing services to the "aging farmer".

Many older adults will be reluctant to move from their home even if remaining is hazardous. Many rural older adults have resided in the same home for most or all of their lives. Their home and land may have been passed down through their family and serve as a strong symbol of their identity. Not only may they have to leave their home, but the lack of available housing in their rural community may force them to move to an unfamiliar area. Older adults often require assistance in relocating to new housing. Special counseling and follow-up services should be provided to all older adults moving to post-disaster housing.

Older rural adults prefer not to have to ask for help, or even acknowledge their need for any disaster services because they view such services as charity. It is helpful to develop an educational program that markets these programs in a way that the local elderly will know how to access services and feel comfortable about doing so. The role of the informal, social support system of the older adult cannot be underestimated, particularly following a disaster. Special efforts may be needed to contact hard-to-reach older adults. In determining long-term needs, it is important to stress flexibility.

Understanding Older People

It has been well documented that people of all ages and cultures reminisce, that is, tell and retell the stories of their lives—whether in the privacy of their own thoughts or in the more public and shared realms of family, friends, community, and media (Campbell, 2002; Webster & McCall, 1999; McAdams, 1993; Bruner, 1990). A consensus on the functions of reminiscing has been more elusive, with thinkers weighing in from a broad range of psychological perspectives (Butler, 1963; Cohler, 1993; Gergen, 1996; Schafer, 1992; Wallace, 1992). Generally, reminiscence is considered a narrative activity in which people conceive and tell stories as a way of making sense of the events that happen to and around them.

Narrative is an ongoing process of meaning-making that is both socially-defined and culturally-grounded. People tend to tell different stories at different times and to different audiences. Webster (1993, 1995, 1997, 1999) proposed eight reasons, or factors, for reminiscing and used them in his Reminiscence Functions Scale (RFS, 1993). These included: Boredom Reduction, Death Preparation, Identity, Problem-Solving, Conversation, Intimacy Maintenance, Bitterness Revival, and Teach/Inform. Campbell (2002) used the RFS to explore the effects on reminiscence functions from clinical depression, specifically in a population of older adults in rural northwestern Illinois. Given that depressed older adults typically experience fatigue/insomnia, anxiety, hopelessness, worthlessness, diminished interest in people and activities, and thoughts of death, Campbell predicted that they would score higher than non-depressed elders on Death Preparation and Bitterness Revival, lower on Conversation and Intimacy Maintenance. Research involving 30 individuals, half of whom had been professionally diagnosed with a significant depressive disorder, demonstrated that the depressed subjects scored significantly higher than their non-depressed peers on Bitterness Revival, with trends toward significance on Boredom Reduction and Identity. No other factor differences were statistically significant. Campbell confirmed that the general tendency within depression to think negatively extends to one's reminiscence. Depressed individuals in this study—more so than their non-depressed peers—identified patterns of reminiscence that frequently focused on painful memories or lost opportunities, and served to fill idle, restless time. No difference appeared in the frequency of overall reminiscence.

Providing Outreach for Older Adults

Linkages should be immediately established with Area Agencies on Aging and Meals on Wheels programs and similar related groups. Networking with local churches is also important. Outreach can be done door-to-door, at senior citizen centers, senior citizen apartments/residential facilities, board and care homes, and trailer and mobile home parks. Services provided should include:

- Home-based counseling
- Services to families and caregivers of older adults
- Older adult support groups
- Video presentations

Such services should be provided at locations convenient for older adults, families, and caregivers. Home-based counseling is often in high demand in rural areas. Older adult support groups have been successful for many communities and provide an opportunity for older disaster survivors to come together and share their fears and worries about the disaster. Video presentations can provide a great opportunity for seniors to come together and discuss their experiences. *Psychosocial Issues for Older Adults in Disasters* (CMHS, 1999) is also an excellent resource.

The following examples demonstrate some other ways to find seniors, family members, or neighbors who may know of rural older adults in need:

Having the experience of adjusting and adapting to the unique circumstances and needs caused by their particular situation, they can often adapt these coping skills and strategies to respond to the challenges of disaster recovery.

An individual who is physically or emotionally challenged may have developed a philosophy that confronts adversity directly. The coping ability of a person who is emotionally challenged is dependent on the support structure surrounding them. The risk to the individual becomes greater when the support structure is also stressed and temporarily or permanently removed. Many such people are also assisted with medications. Following a rural disaster, maintaining or refilling prescriptions can be a significant problem if there is only one local pharmacy and it was damaged or destroyed by the disaster.

People with physical challenges may need to adapt to the environment around them. When that environment undergoes significant change, the person who is physically challenged becomes greatly affected. Accessibility, safety, and autonomy are all diminished, making the person more dependent on the care and assistance of others in responding to the changes brought by the disaster. There may be limited options for transportation. People who are emotionally challenged, depending on their functional level, are often quite capable of managing stress. Rural communities, as well as disruptions in transportation services, can add to the physically challenged person's dependence.

Economically Disadvantaged

Rural poverty levels are often higher than those in urban areas. Some rural individuals and families may have fewer resources. They may not own a home, carry insurance, or have any savings for responding to emergencies. When living from paycheck-to-paycheck, the loss of employment due to disaster places them at great risk.

Economically disadvantaged people are often difficult to locate. A lack of stable employment, living arrangements, and social relationships can make these people a moving target when it comes to outreach. The pre-existing level of need, the present difficulties, and the lack of potential for a very positive outcome all create an almost overwhelming set of needs.

Migrant Farm Workers

Migrant farm workers are often the "hidden" backbone of the farming community's labor pool. They often may be monolingual, difficult to reach, and suspicious of government assistance and intervention. They often reside in "temporary" housing and have limited access to news, radio, or telephones.

An eroding population base in most areas comprises the rural economic outlook. Young adults completing college often do not return to their rural home communities. Social and health service agencies face an increase in demand and a decrease in funding from local and/or State resources.

Under normal circumstances, a scarcity of people, resources, mobility, and support services has characterized rural areas. There is little doubt that rural programs must contend with a more isolated population. However, it can no longer be assumed that geographic isolation means social isolation as well. A farmhouse, a barn, a grain bin, and a satellite dish characterize many farms. Farmers are increasingly "on-line" through computers, connected with universities and other information services. People who live in the country today have daily access to the same information, education, and entertainment options as their urban counterparts.

- High poverty levels
- High unemployment rate
- High levels of social and health related problems
- Pockets of minorities within a largely homogeneous population
- Heavy dependence on agricultural, oil, mining, or tourism related businesses
- Large numbers of people involved with and reliant upon organized religion

Certain community religious groups often emerge as local recovery leaders. For example, in one Midwestern town, the local Methodist minister was also a fire fighter and trained in crisis intervention. He and his wife were both hired as crisis counselors and proved invaluable to the community's recovery and the success of the local crisis counseling project.

Rural Culture and Ethnicity

Cultural and ethnic groups may or may not be identified in great numbers as living in disaster-affected areas. For example, in responding to the Midwest floods, some programs offered services to pockets of groups that required special consideration. A targeted response to African-American, Asian, Hispanic, Native American, and other cultural and ethnic groups was necessary in order for the programs to adequately reach all groups affected by the disaster. Other rural crisis counseling projects served migrant farm workers and homeless individuals.

Even if a rural area appears to be homogeneous, ethnic differences can exist. Differences exist in educational background, religious beliefs, country versus town dwellers, farmers versus ranchers, people who live by the river versus those who do not. Some small communities are as divided along socioeconomic lines of income, education, and religion as are the most diverse inner-city neighborhoods.

In rural areas, ethnic groups may be difficult to find and reach, and gaining their trust may be a challenge. Key community contacts and matching outreach workers to the communities they are to serve can create opportunities for service. Sensitivity to language, traditions, cultural values, and ethics is vital. The rural culture differs from that of urban areas due to the seasonal effect of the work, accessibility, and free time available. Besides the normal phases that people experience after a disaster, there are other timing considerations. In a farming area, times of seeding, ground preparation, and harvest typically offer reduced accessibility of outreach workers to the impacted population. Consideration should also be given to the differing roles and corresponding stressors that apply to men, women, and children in the area. Switching the focus of service delivery to coincide with stress levels and availability may help the program's efficacy overall.

Training in cultural sensitivity should be provided and materials made available in several languages. Workers representative of each local community should be hired, whenever possible, from within each cultural or ethnic group. This helps produce the most successful results. Public information provided in the language preferred and understood by each group increases the likelihood that all people, no matter what their nationality or race, will get the message. It might also be important to use terms and words that are regionally accepted rather than some assumed form of national English.

It is important for a crisis counseling program to reach out to agencies and organizations already known to ethnic and cultural groups. Training staff, providing literature, and interagency collaboration are expected. Consideration should be given to subcontracting service delivery to minority groups or minority-serving agencies. This is often more cost- effective than learning new skills or politicking to overcome barriers.

Four racial and ethnic minority groups — African-Americans, American Indians and Alaska Natives, Asian Americans and Pacific Islanders, and Hispanic Americans — accounted for approximately 30 percent of the U.S. population in the year 2000 and are expected to account for nearly 40 percent or more of the U.S. population by 2025 (DHHS, 2001). Although there are important differences among these four groups, there also is broad diversity within each group. In other words, people who find themselves in the same racial or ethnic group—either by census category or through self-identification—do not always have the same culture. Examples include:

- American Indians and Alaska: Natives may belong to more than 500 tribes, each of which has a different cultural tradition, language, and ancestry (DHHS, 2001).

- Asian Americans and Pacific Islanders may identify with any of 43 subgroups and speak any of 100 languages and dialects (DHHS, 2001).

- Hispanics may be of Mexican, Puerto Rican, Cuban, Central and South American, or other heritage (DHHS, 2001).

Furthermore, the broad category labels are imprecise (DHHS, 2001). For example, people who are indigenous to the Americas may be called Hispanic if they are from Mexico or American Indian if they are from the United States (DHHS, 2001). In addition, many people in a particular racial or ethnic minority group may identify more closely with other social groups than with the group to which they are assigned by definition (DHHS, 2001). Finally, many people identify with multiple cultures that may be associated with factors such as race, ethnicity, country of origin, primary language, immigration status, age, religion, sexual orientation, employment status, disability, geographic location, or socioeconomic status. Recognizing the limitations of the traditional broad groupings, the U.S. Census Bureau revised the categories used to report race and ethnicity in the 2000 Census. For the first time, individuals could identify with more than one group (U.S. Office of Management and Budget, 2000). The U.S. Census Bureau anticipated that this change would result in approximately 63 categories of racial and ethnic identifications (DHHS, 2001).

Cultural Values in Rural Populations

Individualism

A sense of independence and self-determination is more common among residents of rural areas than urban or suburban locations. Many rural residents tend to view themselves and their communities as possessing a higher quality of life and a more realistic, down-to-earth lifestyle than their urban counterparts. Family, close friendships, and a highly developed sense of community, combine to create a sense of self-sufficiency that persists even in the most difficult of circumstances. In times of disaster, these values are often demonstrated as family, friends, and community members provide mutual support, shelter, and care to one another.

Rural people may not actively seek help. They are often not aware of available services or how to access them, or may think the process is too cumbersome or intrusive. Commonly, a farmer or a small business owner may not apply for assistance due to their pride, an underestimation of loss, or a belief that others are more in need of help. If a decision is made to apply for assistance, the process may be particularly difficult for someone unaccustomed to admitting need and seeking assistance. Asking for help is very difficult when the cultural expectation is competence and self-reliance.

Mental Health Stigma

Receiving any form of mental health services may be seen as a negative reflection on a person's character or family life. This attitude can be even more prevalent in rural communities. Disaster survivors may have a negative impression of mental health services and may be offended if made to believe they needed such support. Programming and project identity should avoid the use of mental health jargon. Framing services in terms of disaster survivors deserving counseling services may prove to be more acceptable. Having fewer mental health resources in a community and a self-reliant cultural bias, people in rural communities may lack an understanding of the need and use of mental health services and may benefit from educational presentations about stress management, disaster stress, and coping mechanisms and techniques (NIMH, 1983).

Spiritual Traditions

Some anthropologists and sociologists suggest that all human beings hold some form of spiritual belief. All cultures use spiritual stories, rhetoric, and ritual to find definition for themselves and the world around them. In rural areas, people have a decidedly spiritual quality to the attitudes about natural resources, using land, raising crops or livestock, and living in a community. Rituals surrounding planting and harvest, birth and death, physical and spiritual transformation, patriotism, and loyalty are often embedded in the rural culture.

In rural America, traditional, organized religion is often a powerful exponent of the more basic spiritual values mentioned above. Religious traditions of individuals, families, and communities have become the primary expression of their sense of right and wrong, moral and immoral, good and bad. These traditions provide the structure and language by which they evaluate the world and make decisions.

Spiritual traditions provide the context through which people understand their origin, why they are here, and where they are going. Knowing a person's spiritual context is very important in disaster mental health. Such a personal belief system can aid greatly in the disaster recovery process. In rural communities, churches and other religious institutions provide a valuable resource for finding and serving literally hundreds of people. Collectively, the community they represent is a cross-section of the local social structure with respect to income, education, vocations, and community involvement.

Additional Cultural Considerations

Beyond the fact that rural culture differs from urban culture, there are additional considerations about ethnic cultural differences that need to be taken into account by practitioners who provide services in different rural areas. This is especially important when providing short-term interventions following major disasters, critical incidents, and other crises in a culture not one's own. For example, in Puerto Rico, a United States Commonwealth, some background information is very important. The Estado Libre Asociado de Puerto Rico (autonomous common-wealth), established in 1952, redefined the political relationship between the United States and its colony. The ambiguous political status—autonomy without sovereignty, self-government without self-determination—created new social, political, and cultural contradictions. The island's first elected governor, Luis Munoz Marin, was committed to promoting an essentialized Puerto Rican culture centered around the idealization of traditional rural life, while simultaneously creating a new democratic citizenship, both of which would bolster the new government's legitimacy before its people. Puerto Rican scholar Cati Marsh Kennerley (2003) explored the collective work done by the Division de Educacion de la Comunidad (DivEdCo), the government educational agency charged with promulgating Munoz Marin's ideas about Puerto Rican culture and citizenship. Marsh Kennerley draws from a wide variety of sources to reconstruct an untold history, analyze its contradictions, obtain lessons from DivEdCo's negotiations, and point out its relevance for understanding contemporary Puerto Rican culture. This is important for anyone who will consider providing services in times of need.

In another example, Gavin (2003) shares her experiences of training and working as a psychoanalytical psychotherapist in the United Kingdom and then in a smaller city in the West of Ireland. The range of people seeking counseling and therapy as well as the social arrangements and their effects of the boundaries of the therapy are discussed. Gavin concludes that it is vital to try to understand the cultural context within which one is working but one has to also be clear about what one considers to be the fundamentals of one's particular orientation.

Weyer, Hustey, & Rathbun (2003) provide a case study pertaining to the care of a dying 93-yr-old Amish woman with congestive heart failure living in a rural Amish community. They explore the world of the Amish community in some detail. Their overall beliefs, values, and behavior are discussed as well as how their lifestyle affects their health care decisions, access to health care, and reimbursement of services. Weyer et al state that nurse practitioners can offer culturally sensitive and appropriate healthcare to the Amish population by recognizing important cultural values that have survived for more than 300 years. Such sensitivities are important in understanding and reaching out to other cultural groups effectively.

Phillips, Li, & Zhang (2002) present a picture of the current pattern of suicides in China. Suicide rates by sex, 5-yr age-group, and region (urban or rural) reported by the Chinese Ministry of Health were adjusted according to an estimated rate. It was estimated that a mean annual suicide rate of 23 per 100,000 accounted for 3.6% of all deaths in China and was the fifth most important cause of death for rural women, the eighth most important cause for urban women and men, and the fourteenth most important cause for urban men. The toll was particularly high in individuals aged 15–34 yrs, accounting for 18.9% of such deaths. Rural suicide rates were three times higher in both sexes, for all age-groups, and over time. Suicide is a major health problem for China; this public-health issue demands intervention development for high-risk persons. A number of different explanations are likely plausible for such high rates. Reardon (2002) suggests that the uniquely high rates documented by Phillips et al may be partly explained by the strictly enforced birth quotas in China while Bertolote and Fleischmann (2002) point out the association between suicide and mental disorders.

Customs and Traditions for Healing

Many cultural groups hold beliefs about illness and healing that differ sharply from those held by the Western cultures. People in every culture share beliefs about the causes of illness and ideas about how suffering can be mitigated. For example, members of some cultures believe that physical and emotional problems result from spiritual wrongdoings in this life or a previous one. They believe that healing requires forgiveness from ancestors or higher spirits. Some people believe that suffering cannot be alleviated (DeVries, 1996). Others demonstrate stress and emotional conflict through complaints about their physical health. Traditional healers, such as local herbalists, faith healers, Curanderos, and acupuncturists, play important roles in recovery of mental and physical health within some cultures. In general, the work of healers is based on the principle that the body cannot be isolated from the mind, and the mind cannot be removed from its social context. Disaster mental health workers who interact with cultures in which healers play a key role in health must understand the concepts of integration of body, mind, and spirit when they provide disaster crisis counseling services to diverse populations. They must be able to integrate traditional methods of healing into service delivery (de Monchy, 1991). Although the crisis counselor may not subscribe to certain cultural healing beliefs, he or she must acknowledge their existence and recognize their importance to some disaster survivors. At the same time, the worker must be alert for any use of dangerous healing practices, such as ingestion of harmful mixtures containing lead or other toxic substances, and take corrective measures. Reestablishing rituals in appropriate locations is another way to help survivors in the recovery process. Symbolic gathering places, such as churches, mosques, trees, and safe places for meeting after sundown, are important in some cultures and are required for certain rituals.

After a disaster, survivors may lose access to symbolic places, and this loss may limit their ability to mobilize healing resources. Identifying new locations for rituals can foster social support and facilitate coping mechanisms following disaster (DeVries, 1996). Disaster mental health workers also may help organize culturally appropriate anniversary activities and commemorations as a way to help survivors mark a milestone in the healing process. Cultural and religious traditions, including special ways of both celebrating and mourning, can be incorporated into such events and may enrich their symbolic meaning and healing potential. Any attempts to facilitate activities involving customs and traditions must be undertaken carefully and only after consultation with members of the involved cultural groups.

Rural psychology has very few major studies concerning practice in rural environments and small communities. Practitioners face some very different problems from their more urban counterparts. Rural practice presents important yet challenging issues for mental health, especially given the North American and international distribution of the population, levels of need for mental health services in rural settings, limited availability of rural services, and migration of rural residents to urban centers. Direct service issues include the need to accommodate a wide variety of mental health difficulties, issues related to client privacy and boundaries, and practical challenges. Indirect service issues include the greater need for diverse professional activities, including collaborative work with professionals having different orientations and beliefs, program development and evaluation, and conducting research with few mentors or peer collaborators. Professional training and development issues include lack of specialized relevant courses and placements, and such personal issues as limited opportunities for recreation and culture, and lack of privacy. Mental Health will need to address more fully these complex issues if rural residents are to receive equitable treatment and services (Barbopoulos & Clark, 2003).

Grief: A Brief Cross-Cultural Perspective

Cultural beliefs can be both resources and barriers in providing support for grieving families. Across cultures, people differ in what they believe and understand about life and death, what they feel, what elicits those feelings, the perceived implications of those feelings, the ways they express those feelings, the appropriateness of certain feelings, and the techniques for dealing with feelings that cannot be directly expressed (Rosenblatt, 1993). Historical studies have shown how individuals in western cultures have mourned differently over time (Newnes, 1991; Kohn & Levav, 1990). A cross-cultural perspective shows an infinite variety in people's responses to death, in how they mourn, and in the nature of their internalization of the lost object. Rather than being process-oriented, mourning is seen as an adaptive response to specific task demands arising from loss that must be dealt with regardless of individual, culture, or historical era (Hagman, 1995).

Americans report thinking significantly more about grief, religious feelings, and death than do Japanese (Asai & Barnlund, 1998). Ancestor worship in Japan is ritual. It is supported by a sophisticated theory through which the living manage their bonds with the dead. It is a process similar to the resolution of grief in the modern west (Klass, 1996). Klass & Heath (1997) explored the grief of Japanese parents after abortion and the ritual by which the grief is resolved. The ritual is Mizuko Ruyo. Mizuko means "child of the water". Ruyo is a Buddhist offering. In a ritual drama played out by Jizo, the bodhisattva who suffers for others, the parents' pain and the child's pain are connected. In that connection, the pain of each is resolved. The child is made part of the community and does not become a spirit bringing harm to the family. The parents can fulfill their obligation to care for the child and transform the sense of *kurnon*, sickness unto death, into a realization of Buddhism's first noble truth, i.e. that all life is suffering. In a slightly different cultural context, *The Bardo Thodol* (Tibetan Book of the Dead) together with its associated ritual provides a way to understand how Buddhism in Tibetan culture manages the issues associated with what is called grief in Western psychology. The resolution of grief in the survivors is intertwined with the journey to the rebirth of the deceased (Goss & Klass, 1997).

The primary mental health benefits of ritual are closely tied to the relational aspects of the ritual process. These act to validate and encourage the healthy expression of a wide range of human emotions. Jacobs (1992) concludes that religious ceremony and ritual functions mitigate anxiety and deal effectively with other problematic emotional states. Religious rites have a cathartic effect as emotions are released and expressed through attachment and connection to significant others. Reeves (1989, 1990) suggests that ritual can be used to assist individuals to move from a maladaptive to an adaptive style of grieving.

Rubin (1990) used social network theory to compare mourning behaviors in the United States with those in Israeli kibbutz. He found that in a dense social network, such as a small or medium-sized kibbutz, mourning is part of a wider circle of family, friends, neighbors, and co-workers. He suggests that the funerals in the United States may force loose social networks to generate an image of social support. Rubin suggests using social network theory as a basis for cross-cultural analysis of the range of participation in mourning rituals.

Hagman (1995) reviewed the standard psychoanalytic model of mourning and suggests that the model may not be generally valid. The psychoanalytic literature and data from clinical practice fail to confirm basic components of mourning theory. Stroebe (1992,1993) challenges the belief in the importance of "grief work" for adjustment to bereavement (the grief work hypothesis). She examined claims made in theoretical formulations and principles of grief counseling and therapy concerning the necessity of working through loss. Reviews of empirical evidence and cross-cultural findings document alternative patterns of coping with grief. Stroebe argues that there are grounds for questioning a grief hypothesis.

Existing definitions and operationalizations are problematic. The few empirical studies that have examined the impact of grief work have yielded equivocal results Grief work is not a universal concept. She proposes a revision of the definition of grief work, which overcomes the confounding of the process with symptomatology and should facilitate future empirical testing, and suggests a differential approach.

Teams of counselors dispatched to mass casualty disaster sites can, at times, be an overwhelming presence. Sensitivity to cultural needs and desires are necessary to provide appropriate and desired services. Newell (1998), in a cross-cultural study of privacy, found that the majority of students (aged 17–45) from Ireland, Senegal, and the United States in their study believed that not being disturbed was the most important element of privacy and grief. Fatigue and the need to focus were the main affective sets associated with seeking privacy. The affect associated with a desire for privacy, the definition of privacy as a condition of the person, the duration of the average privacy experience, and the change in affect at the completion of the experience suggested that privacy has a therapeutic effect.

In summary, sensitivity to the culturally appropriate needs for ritual in responding to grief and providing for privacy and personal needs are paramount. Imposing a "one size fits all" grief model on people, however well-intentioned, may cause more harm and ill feeling than good. Respect for the beliefs, rituals and desires of those affected can accomplish far more than unwanted attention and interventions.

In reaching all community members, some programs develop flyers explaining common disaster reactions with a phone number for more information. Placing them in grocery bags at check-out stands, posting on community bulletin boards, and distributing at banks provide additional outlets for information and outreach

It is important to remember the power of the pulpit. Religious leaders can provide background information at sermons. Offer religious organizations inserts for church/synagogue/mosque programs and bulletins, flyers for bulletin boards, and coloring pages for children.

Cross-Cultural Counseling and Psychotherapy

The powerful thrust toward the development of comprehensive mental health services throughout the world has stimulated the search for a way to integrate the services already there, indigenous and available, with those of the imported variety.

Within the last few decades, a body of writing has come into being dealing with the delivery of mental health services beyond cultural frontiers (Higginbotham, 1976, 1979a, 1979b). The World Health Organization has been engaged in a project in four developing countries around the world—Columbia, India, Sudan, and Senegal—on the development of community-based mental health services (Diop, Collignon, and Gueye, 1976). In these efforts, blending in of native psychotherapy is an important component.

Indigenous psychotherapy refers to the whole range of verbal and inter-personal techniques, designed for the alleviation of personal distress and for the induction of change of behavior, which have been developed independently of the Western tradition of scientifically based psychotherapy (Draguns, 1981). Both psychotherapy and counseling function to alleviate distress, to reintegrate the client or patient into the culture, and to enable him or her to respond to cultural roles and to meet cultural expectations (Draguns, 1981).

Briefly, it may be helpful at this point to define what is meant in this paper by the terms counseling and psychotherapy. Counseling is an activity that facilitates and fosters personal problem solving. Psychotherapy is principally concerned with changing persons, their characteristic modes of subjective experience and overt behavior—that is, their personalities (Draguns, 1981).

A major share of the literature in this field is devoted to the maladaptation and stress of the culture contact situation. The problems of people removed from their cultural roots, through migration, sojourn, or involuntary displacement, occupy the efforts of a great many culturally-oriented mental health professionals (Alexander, Klein, Miller, and Workneh, 198; Pedersen, Lonner, and Draguns, 1976; Taft, 1977). This is also true about the phenomenon of culture shock. There is a considerable amount of information which has come into being on how to help people who are casualties of intercultural mobility. Examples include distraught college students, confused immigrants, traumatized expellees and refugees, and discouraged and dissatisfied Peace Corps volunteers. There have been attempts to sketch a composite portrait of an individual who is least or most likely to succumb to this kind of stress (Pinter, 1969). Characteristics of host environments have also been scrutinized in attempts to identify those features which contribute to making such an environment particularly stressful or unusually stress-free for newcomers (Taft, 1977).

There is a sizeable amount of literature which deals with psychotherapy and counseling with individuals who have been transplanted to a new cultural setting (Szapocznik, Scopetta, Arondale, and Kurtines, 1978; David, 1976). This body of writing provides practical relevant information for the professional involved in extending services to immigrants, sojourners, or returnees from intensive cross-cultural encounters such as Peace Corps Volunteers.

In highly controlled and over-regulated environments, psychotherapy may provide an avenue of release for feelings and emotions, a sort of safety valve (Tseng and Hsu, 1979). In contrast, in an under-regulated or even perhaps an anomic setting, psychotherapy would be likely to emphasize external and social control at the expense of self-expression. These two formulations open the possibility for testing differential hypotheses. This is a task which has not yet been attempted.

There have been statements made about the relationship of these impressionistic differences to the dominant values and the official ideologies of the countries in question (Wittkower and Warnes, 1974). The parallel between the prevalence of authoritarian-totalitarian political regimes and the de-emphasis of exploratory, open-minded, insight-oriented therapy has repeatedly been noted in Germany, Japan, and the Soviet Union (Draguns, 1981). Two of these countries have experienced an abrupt change in their political orientation, with a considerable cultural change in its wake. It has been suggested that in the United States, however, the goals and the ethos of psychotherapy have been transformed as the values in the larger society have changed.

In Japan, the two indigenously developed therapies, Naikan and Morita, are based on guilt induction and control and on suppression of communication respectively. In the Naikan system, the client is admonished to think of all the ways in which he has wronged his/her mother (Tanaka-Matsumi, 1979). In the course of Morita therapy, what the client may say, and when and how, is elaborately restricted and ritualized (Reynolds, 1976). The contrast between Western expectations and Japanese therapy is stark. Documentation on Morita therapy indicates that this therapy works in a substantial proportion of cases on its home grounds. As Sue (1977) has pointed out, therapy and counseling services geared to a culturally distinct group have to be appropriate in process and in goals to be acceptable and effective.

Across cultures, there is much of value to learn from indigenous therapies. As Torrey (1972b) has put it, we have something to learn from the witch doctors. What we as modern psychotherapists and counselors could learn from them is to separate the effective ingredients from the incidental trappings in our own implementation of therapeutic services. Probably, for as long as psychotherapy and counseling have been practiced, these services have been delivered. In some instances, at least, they have even been delivered across cultural lines. An example is Freud's (1953) treatment of the "wolf-man". Erikson (1950) drew upon therapeutic and quasi-therapeutic situations beyond the mainstream of American culture. Seward (1956) illustrated her work on culture and personality with case studies of psychotherapy with Americans from a variety of cultural backgrounds. Abel (1956) addressed the problem of the role of cultural factors among American clients in psychotherapy. Devereux (1951, 1953) ventured beyond the usual settings in which psychotherapy was conducted in order to undertake, and to report in detail, psychoanalytically-oriented psychotherapy with a "Plains Indian". The person was not further identified in terms of nation or tribe in order to protect his privacy.

All of the above early contributions have extended verbal psychotherapy to new groups of clients, demonstrated its effectiveness on the case level with new populations, and illustrated the serendipitous "fallout" of psychotherapy as an avenue of learning about the personal experience of another culture. Currently, there are approaches which are even more venturesome and that involve not only the extension but the adaptation of the therapy technique and experience as well.

All people respond to stimuli and situations by either changing themselves or the environment and by combining these two operations in various proportions. Particularly, psychotherapy with international students was characterized in the past by facilitating the process of accommodation to, and acceptance of, the host's culture norms. The possibility of extending the individual's scope of choices in the service of actively changing the environment was neglected and underemphasized. Historically, the implicit goal of counseling and psychotherapy has been to bring about a greater degree of conformity to the norms of the dominant majority group. In the case of members of minority groups, the contemporary counselor or therapist faces a choice. The therapist can prepare the client for changing obstacles in the environment, or he can equip him or her for a greater degree of accommodation to the social structure in its current state. In a pluralistic society like the United States, the increase in the individual's options also involves choices on the nature and extent of one's relationships, reference groups, and identity, especially in relation to one's ethnic or cultural group.

Wrenn (1962) sensitized counselors to the problem of cultural encapsulation and warned against the imposition of culturally alien goals, values, and practices upon clients across cultural lines. Pedersen (1976) has taken the position that, at least in the multicultural setting of the United States, crossing the cultural gulf in the mental health field is the rule rather than the exception. Extending the concept of culture, he has maintained that the cultures of the counselor and of the counselee may be expected to differ—slightly, yet perceptibly—in most counseling encounters.

Developments, such as those mentioned, resulted in recommendations made at the Vail Conference on Clinical Psychology, which was sponsored by the American Psychological Association (Korman, 1974). The knowledge of the cultures of one's clients has been elevated to an ethical imperative. As a result, doing therapy or counseling without cultural sensitivity, knowledge, or awareness is not just problematic, it has been declared unethical. The implication of these recommendations is that the knowledge on therapy and culture has ceased being an esoteric field. It has, instead, become a matter of direct and practical concern for the vast majority of clinical and counseling psychologists in the pluralistic culture of the United States.

The problems of doing research across cultural lines can be overwhelming. Much has been said about variations in psychotherapy around the world constituting a laboratory of nature. The existing literature on cultural variations of psychotherapy pertains, with a few exceptions, to cultural variations in the United States. Abramowitz and Dokecki's (1977) review, based on analogue studies, seems to corroborate the impression that, in the appraisal of individuals in the mental health setting at this time, in the United States, class lines exercise a greater effect upon the interviewer than do race and sex.

Draguns (1981) suggests that four kinds of information are needed in research across cultural lines:

- Intracultural data on the effects and consequences of various indigenous therapy techniques
- Cross-cultural comparisons of effectiveness of various techniques of psychotherapy, varying and, in the ideal case, counterbalancing both culture and psychotherapeutic technique

- Comparing the effectiveness of indigenous and extraneous psychotherapies in a given setting.

- Since native components of psychotherapy are increasingly being utilized, from Lambo's (1962; Erinsho, 1976) village model to the use of traditional healers within the Hispanic populations of North American cities (Ruiz and Longrod, 1976), the effect of using these indigenous mental health specialists upon the outcome should be investigated.

Does the addition of healers of one's own cultural tradition result in the enhancement of effectiveness of mental health services? A start has been made in investigating the efficacy of Morita Therapy (Miura and Usa, 1970; Reynolds, 1976) and Naikan Therapy (Tanaka-Matsumi, 1979) in Japan. These are two procedures indigenous to their culture, yet developed and practiced by modern mental health professionals.

Jilek-Aal (1978) has noted the effectiveness of the Salish Indian spirit dance in promoting therapeutic change in alcoholics and other patients of that cultural group. It induces regression through an altered state of consciousness, promotes the experience of death and rebirth, and provides the participant with a new identity reoriented toward the ideal of the Salish culture. The rationale and the procedure appear to be reminiscent of the fixed-role therapy of George Kelly (1955), except for the greater reliance on affective and regressive processes, and on altered states of consciousness.

One of the things that therapists of diverse orientations and cultures share is the ability to generate perceptions of competence and concern in their clients (Torrey, 1972b). The therapist's role, regardless of technique, is catalytic. He enables the client to make use of his or her existing assets and strengths (Prince, 1976, 1980). Non-western cultures have tended to rely to a greater extent than the west upon the induction of altered states of consciousness to bring about these catalytic effects. The range of such techniques is wide. What is lacking at this point is a more explicit, systematic, and specific understanding of what techniques fulfill what expectations on the basis of what kinds of culturally-mediated learning.

On the negative side, psychotherapy fosters dependency, disorganization, passivity, and non-spontaneity (Mendel, 1972). In terms of concrete operations, the universals in psychotherapy include confrontation, exploration of the past, exploring new alternative behaviors, and trying them out in practice. While Torrey (1972a, 1972b) and Prince (1976, 1980) address themselves to the issue of what matters in psychotherapy, Mendel (1972) is principally concerned with the problem of what happens in psychotherapy.

What features of a culture are reflected in its therapeutic services? What kinds of models are implicitly emulated in the conduct of psychotherapy? Once again, one can only point to statements placing psychotherapy in its respective cultural context (Draguns, 1975; Neki, 1973; Wittkower and Warnes, 1974) and relating it to the needs, expectations, models, and opportunities experienced in that culture.

Collomb (1973) has attempted to answer the question: What impels a mental health professional to offer services outside his or her usual geographic and cultural milieu, and how may these motives interfere with his or her optimal functioning as a therapist? He has presented a provisional typology of what might be called the cultural distortions of countertransference. On the basis of his observations, he has distinguished three attitudes that could be described as those of universalism, cultural uniqueness, and rejection of one's own culture of origin.

One prerequisite with which it is difficult to disagree is that the therapist, as part of his/her expertise and competence, should know the culture within which he/she operates. Deveraux (1969), for example, applied himself to a thorough study of the "Plains Indians", preparatory and concurrent to conducting psychotherapy with one of them.

In reference to a great many American ethnic groups, Giordano and Giordano (1976) have provided valuable and specific information that the counselor or therapist should keep in mind in initiating and maintaining contacts with members of these groups. It would be a grave mistake to do psychotherapy in the same way with all the people designated African-American, Mexican, or American Indian. Yet, the knowledge of the culture of one's clients provides the therapist with an entree and/or point of departure. The therapist's experience with a cultural group or the information on it in the relevant professional literature serves as a source of hypotheses, to be verified, discarded and modified on the basis of information acquired in the course of psychotherapy.

Therapists undertaking to treat members of minority groups should approach this task with a maximum of self-awareness and be prepared to deal with their own distortions of the therapy experience and relationship. An important theme that pervades the literature is the importance of client-therapist compatibility. The most concrete, but perhaps the most crucial, form that this compatibility takes is for both the therapist and the client to be members of the same minority group.

What emerges as a common thread in the writings of therapy with African-Americans, Mexican Americans, American Indians, and Asian Americans is the independent emphasis that writers of various persuasions and orientations place on activity, as opposed to reflection and passivity, as the recommended mode of intervention with these several groups (Abad, Ramos, and Boyce, 1974; Atkinson, Maruyama, and Matsui, 1978; Banks, Berenson, and Carkhuff, 1967; Peoples and Dell, 1975; Ruiz and Padilla, 1977; Smith, 1977; Sue and Sue, 1972; Sue and McKinney, 1975; Vontress, 1969, 1970).

Weidman (1975), in her work with members of other cultures in Miami, Florida, pioneered the concept of culture-broker, a well-informed intermediary whose inputs are brought to bear upon the therapy process. Least formally and most ubiquitously, the client remains the major source of information about those features of his or her cultural experience which might otherwise baffle the therapist. The limit of this mode of inquiry is that the individual, not the culture, is the focus of all therapy (Draguns, 1981). Sessions should not deteriorate into ethnographic data-gathering in its own right and for its own purpose, nor to satisfy the therapist's curiosity. Rather, the referent should be: is this information needed for therapy, and, if so, how?

Rural Practice

Jensen & Royeen (2002) describe the processes and outcomes of an action research project targeted at describing 'best practice' as experienced by interdisciplinary rural health projects funded by the Quentin N. Burdick Program for Rural Interdisciplinary Training, a Federally funded training grant competition in the USA. Each of 15 rural interdisciplinary health training projects across the areas of mental health, chronic disease, diabetes, minority health, and geriatrics was used to build a qualitative case study representing best practice experiences in projects focused on improving rural access to care. Across these programs, best practice is seen in the integrated dimensions of connections, community, and culture. In the USA, academic institutions build meaningful, authentic connections with rural communities as they work together in meeting community needs, while demonstrating sensitivity and respect for cultural perspectives. Implications are offered in the context of higher education, healthcare delivery, and Federal initiatives within the USA.

Not only does the culture of rurality have differences from that of urban areas, but rural cross-cultural differences are also important in understanding and providing appropriate responses and services to residents of rural environments. Further attention and study of these areas as well as the awareness of what is already known is needed to inform mental health and other professionals working in these areas.

Arguing that, if done right, ranching has the power to restore ecological integrity to American western lands, Knight (Editor), Gilgert , and Marston (2002) present essays, anecdotes, and a few poems that address the state of the rancher and suggest ways to improve the practice of ranching in view of today's realities. The essayists attack what they perceive as the two enemies of ranching, the developers of suburban subdivisions and Wal-Marts, as well as over-zealous environmentalists who "see cows as the source of all evil". The essayists also address the failures of ranchers themselves, suggesting at various times that ranchers must get used to a marginal economic existence, must interact more with urban environments and peoples, and must steward the ecosystems of their lands with greater care.

The book *Ranching West of the 100th Meridian* offers a literary and thought-provoking look at ranching and its role in the changing West. Its lyrical and deeply felt narratives, combined with fresh information and analysis, offer a poignant and enlightening consideration of ranchers' ecological commitments to the land, their cultural commitments to American society, and the economic role ranching plays in sustainable food production and the protection of biodiversity.

The book begins with writings that bring to life the culture of ranching, including the fading reality of families living and working together on their land, generation after generation. The middle section offers an understanding of the ecology of ranching, from issues of overgrazing and watershed damage to the concept that grazing animals can actually help restore degraded land. The final section addresses the economics of ranching in the face of declining commodity prices and rising land values brought by the increasing suburbanization of the West.

Livestock ranching in the West has been attacked from all sides—by environmentalists who see cattle as a scourge upon the land, by fiscal conservatives who consider the leasing of grazing rights to be a massive federal handout program, and by developers who covet intact ranches for subdivisions and shopping centers. The authors acknowledge that, if done wrong, ranching clearly has the capacity to hurt the land. But if done right, it has the power to restore ecological integrity to Western lands that have been too-long neglected. *Ranching West of the 100th Meridian* makes a unique and impassioned contribution to the ongoing debate on the future of the New West.

Rural Emergency Services

The attributes of the rural setting, the emergency psychiatric services, the staff, the patients, and a program to meet these needs are described by Bassuk & Cote (1983). They distributed a questionnaire to directors of the emergency service of each community mental health center in Vermont in 1979. Results suggest that the extensive informal network of crisis care providers gives rural emergency services their unique character.

Hospitals

Psychologists work in many different domains within the rural hospital environment, but their services in the rural hospital emergency room may be the most critical. As Morris (1997) emphasizes, medical emergencies frequently have significant behavioral and psychological components that require psychologists' knowledge-base, assessment, consultation, crisis intervention, and treatment skills to respond fully to the needs of patients and their families. Morris concludes that the psychologist and physician make an especially powerful combination in the rural healthcare environment.

Hessen (1989) discusses the psychosocial support provided by a psychiatric outpatient clinic at a small rural hospital in Norway in connection with a plane crash that produced 36 casualties. The disaster training of human service workers, psychiatric emergency plans, emotional support, cooperation between health and social services, long-term support functions, use of the media, responsibility for support work, use of experts on psychosocial intervention in crisis work, and work routines for and psychological debriefing of psychiatric personnel were areas found to be of significance in handling the situation.

Schools

Crises in schools take on a number of different aspects at various levels. Critical incidents, such as Columbine High School massacre, tend to receive greater attention, especially in the media. However, there are also other areas of group and individual crisis that, if addressed early enough, could possibly help prevent greater crises or incidents later (Rose-Gold (1991).

Planning and Response

Peoples' reactions to disaster and their coping skills, as well as their receptivity to crisis counseling, differ significantly because of their individual beliefs, cultural traditions, and economic and social status in their community. In order to respond effectively to the mental health needs of all disaster survivors, crisis counseling programs need to be sensitive to the unique experiences, beliefs, norms, values, traditions, customs, and language of each individual, regardless of his or her racial, ethnic, or cultural background. Disaster mental health services must be provided in a manner that recognizes, respects, and builds on the strengths and resources of survivors and their communities. It is critical to assist States and communities in planning, designing, and implementing culturally competent disaster mental health services for survivors of natural and human-caused disasters of all scales.

The ongoing threat of both natural and human-caused disasters makes it imperative to support and encourage the brave men and women who prepare for and respond to these events—our crisis response professionals. These professionals include first responders, public health workers, construction workers, transportation workers, utilities workers, volunteers, and a multitude of others. The focus needs to be on general principles of stress management. It should offer simple, practical strategies that can be incorporated into the daily routine of managers and workers and also provide a concise orientation to the signs and symptoms of stress.

Crisis counseling program services are best accomplished when there is an existing plan in place for:

- rapid mobilization

- response

- implementation of disaster mental health services

Does your State and local department of mental health have a mental health disaster plan? Is the plan a component of the State and local emergency management plan?

Culture changes continuously. For example, immigrants to the United States bring with them their own beliefs, norms, and values, but through the process of acculturation they gradually learn and adopt selected elements of the dominant culture. An immigrant group may develop its own culture while becoming acculturated. At the same time, the dominant culture may change as a result of its interaction with the immigrant group (DHHS, 2001).

Culture is not static. Rather, it is a dynamically changing entity. We influence other cultures, and other cultures influence us. Chinese and Asian medicine has become part of the American and European health cultures. Silver & Wilson (1988) have used American Indian purification and healing practices in the treatment of PTSD. In Bergen, for example, a remote part of the world, we may have our own shaman, influenced by African practices. We should be aware of how we can influence cultural change, but not be afraid to try to make a difference when aspects of a prevailing culture negatively affect children, nor should we adopt cultural practices uncritically. But at the same time, we need to be very aware of the relativity of what we look upon as negative aspects of a culture. We should continue to improve our research methods, scrutinize our findings, and be open to new therapeutic advances; but we should never forget that history repeatedly has shown us that we, as adults, have overlooked, disregarded, and denied the pain and suffering of children.

For those residing in rural and isolated parts of Canada, obtaining quality mental health services is often an unfulfilled wish. Rural and isolated communities share the problems of health status and access to care. Health deteriorates the greater the distance from urban areas in the following dimensions:

- Lower life expectancy than the national average
- Higher rates of disability
- Violence
- Poisoning
- Suicide and accidental death
- More mental and physical health issues than those who live in urban areas

The Canadian Collaborative Mental Health Initiative (CCMHI) was formed to provide, in part, a practical means to encouraging collaborations between primary care and mental health providers.

Lessons Learned

Key messages from the consultative process included: access to services, inter-professional education, consumer involvement, research and evaluation, models of collaboration, ethics, funding, and policy and legislation. A flow diagram was devised to detail the synthesis and practical application of the toolkit, as well as the challenges, key questions and principles of implementation associated with collaborative care initiatives in rural and isolated regions.

The client remains the major source of information about those features of his or her cultural experience which might otherwise baffle the therapist. The limit of this mode of inquiry is that the individual, not the culture, is the focus of all therapy. In cross-cultural counseling and psychotherapy, an attempt is made to deal with the individual within the context of his or her cultural milieu, and to adapt and adjust to it effectively. When they live in an alien or new culture, the problem of adjusting to two cultures complicates the task.

3 Disaster Mental Health in Rural Areas

Background

Crises in the form of individual events, critical incidents, and disasters occur in rural and frontier areas of America just as they do elsewhere. They do have effects on people, and events elsewhere have effects as well. These may occur vicariously (e.g. video reports and pictures from September 11 or hostages in Iraq) and/or they may happen to family, friends, or colleagues. Some of the crises that can, and do, occur in rural areas include the crises of war, suicide, school problems, domestic violence, vicarious trauma, and disasters (e.g., fires, floods, earthquakes, technological disasters, hurricanes, and tornadoes and their effects in rural environments).

Conditions in the West and ranching culture, including the rural geography, the cowboy mystique, the social fabric of the rural lifestyle, and the "health" of agriculture can negatively impact the delivery of rural health services and the attitude of ranchers and farmers toward seeking help for personal problems. These conditions may create a behavioral hazard to ranchers, farmers, and individuals in the West. It is important to understand and develop strategies that exist to improve the availability and acceptance of rural behavioral health services.

Emergency crews in rural areas face certain challenges that urban crews may not. These challenges center mainly around the fact that people in small communities tend to know each other and that many emergency workers are volunteers who give up time with their families to work in the service of their communities.

The mental health component of disaster relief was incorporated in Public Law 93-288 in the 1970s and mandated the National Institute of Mental Health to provide counseling services and training materials. Much attention has been devoted to this over the years. However, studies have shown that small rural communities require a different kind of attention because of their unique characteristics (Farberow, 1985). These include pride in independence, rejection of the unfamiliar, a tendency to take problems to family rather than professionals, a larger number of persons living well below the poverty line, and less acceptance of mental illness.

Typical Disasters Affecting Rural Areas

There are many types of disasters and crises that occur in rural areas. Some are small and individual in impact, whereas others affect much larger populations.

Fires

In September 1991, in the small rural town of Hamlet, NC, a fryer exploded at a chicken-processing plant, killing 25 employees and injuring many more. This disaster stirred national attention, influenced state laws and inspection policies, and profoundly affected the entire community. Derosa (1995) examined the relationship between PTSD and the survivors' subjective experiences of the trauma, their search for meaning, and their perceptions of self, of others, and of the world around them. They attempted to capture the survivor's experiences of themes such as rage, grief, and a belief in a benevolent world. They did this in conjunction with clinical diagnoses of PTSD (using the SCID interview) in order to assess the buffering or exacerbating influence on subjective experiences. Seventy-eight subjects included plant employees, relatives of employees, rescue personnel, and relatives of fire/rescue personnel. Several categories of variables were examined. These included unresolved trauma themes, 'pre-fire' variables—including neuroticism, history of traumatic experiences, and previous psychiatric treatment—'peri-traumatic' variable—including dissociation, fear of injury, and level of exposure to the fire—as well as types of social support, and demographics.

The most robust variables contributing to lifetime diagnosis of PTSD after the fire were: having lower socio-economic status, being female, feeling little social support, fearing death/injury, and dissociating during the fire. The only significant contribution to the model for chronic PTSD was the number of unresolved trauma themes. Additionally, the degree to which the trauma themes remained maladaptive varied by the severity of diagnosis. Exploratory cluster analyses of patterns of unresolved themes among survivors and their families suggested that in addition to the number of unresolved themes, the pattern of thematic resolution was associated with diagnosis.

Eyles, Taylor, & Baxter (1993) studied the 1990 Hagersville (Ontario) tire fire. They described the accounts of 43 residents affected by the fire, evacuation, and aftermath in terms of concerns, anxieties, and responses. Five themes emerged: economic, community, health, environmental, and governance.

Floods

In June 1981, south-eastern Kentucky experienced serious and widespread flooding. In May 1984, a storm system brought tornadoes, strong winds, and severe, extensive flooding to this same area. What impact did these two floods have upon the mental, physical, and social functioning of the rural Appalachian victims? Were these individuals able to take these events 'in stride' or did they present a serious challenge to their ability to cope? Did these floods leave a lasting impact upon the mental and physical well-being of these individuals or did they only result in relatively minor and short-lived emotional upset? Were some people more affected than others? Were these communities able to 'rally around' their members or were they shattered and split apart? These questions and others were the focus of a study of the psychosocial impact of the Kentucky floods by Norris, Phifer, & Kaniasty (1994). This study had three features that hold particular promise for increasing what we know about the effects of disaster:

1. the study's prospective and longitudinal design
2. its consideration of both individual and collective aspects of disaster exposure
3. its focus on older people (aged 55 or older)

In another study of flood victims, Ginexi, Weihs, & Simmens (2000) examined whether the 1993 Midwest floods increased depression symptoms and diagnoses in a statewide sample of 1,735 Iowa residents (aged 18-90 yrs), approximately half of whom were victims of the 1993 floods. The residents participated in interviews one year prior to, and thirty to ninety days after, the disaster. Employing a rigorous methodology, including both control-group comparisons and pre-disaster assessments, Ginexi et al performed a systematic evaluation of the disaster's impact. Overall, the disaster led to true but small rises in depressive symptoms and diagnoses 60–90 days post-flood. The disaster-psychopathology effect was not moderated by pre-disaster depressive symptoms or diagnostically defined depression. Instead, pre-disaster symptoms and diagnoses uniquely contributed to increases in post-disaster distress. However, increases in symptoms as a function of impact were slightly greater among respondents with the lowest incomes and among residents living in small rural communities, as opposed to on farms or in cities.

Sundet & Mermelstein (1996) examined why some survived the Great Flood of 1993 in the Midwest and others did not, and the relationship of those outcomes to classic crisis intervention theory. Qualitative case investigations were conducted from eight severely impacted river towns in Missouri. Graduate social work students began on-site data gathering approximately seven weeks after the flood's initial strike in the state. Results suggested that specific, pre-disaster community characteristics were associated with post-disaster survival or failure. Among demographic variables, only the poverty rate appeared to have a strong association with outcome. Contrary to expectations, a vibrant economy was not a predictor of community survival. Communication skills, on the other hand, were invaluable aids in survival.

Following floods in France in 1996, Maltais, Lachance, & Brassard (2002) studied qualitative and quantitative problems and emotions experienced by 122 male and female adults (mean age 48.4 yrs)—victims of floods in rural areas—and 117 male and female adults living in an area unaffected by the flooding. Data on socio-demographic variables and physical, social, and mental symptoms experienced during the emergency phase and the recovery process were obtained by semi-structured interviews, conducted three years after the flood. The Impact of Event Scale (M. J. Horowitz et al, 1979), the Beck Depression Inventory, the General Health Questionnaire, and the Affect Balance Scale (N. M. Bradburn, 1969) were used. The results suggest that the health status was more delicate and financial situations more unstable among subjects affected by the flood than among those subjects not affected by the flood. This information has implications for developing intervention methods for victims of natural disasters.

Solomon & Smith (1994) discuss the impact of exposure to flooding and/or dioxin contamination on rural St. Louis residents experiencing these events in late 1982. This study was designed to describe the type and extent of psychiatric disturbance that followed these events, and to see if victims' reactions varied for the different types of disasters. They were also interested in learning how social support and family role affected victims' reactions and which victims were most likely to experience psychological problems following exposure. They explored why some people react more negatively to both disaster exposure and the lack of social support than do others. Toward this end, they explored perceived control as a possible explanation of victims' responses to disaster.

In summary, poverty levels, general economic conditions, perceived control, previous experience, and rurality all seem to have effects on responses and recovery and psychosocial adjustments from flooding disasters. These and other variables need to be considered when planning for post-disaster interventions and responses in rural environments.

Earthquakes

Wang, Gao, & Zhang (2000) examined longitudinal change of quality of life (QOL) and psychological wellbeing in a community sample affected by an earthquake and examined the relationship between QOL and disaster exposure, post-disaster support and other related variables. The Ss, from two villages at different distances from the epicenter, were assessed using the brief version of the World Health Organization Quality of Life Assessment (WHOQOL-BREF) and three subscales of a symptoms checklist at three months (n = 335) and nine months (n = 253) after the earthquake, respectively. Exposure to the earthquake was associated with multidimensional impairment in QOL, including physical, psychological and environmental domains at three months, and psychological and environmental domains at nine months. The victims also suffered significantly more psychological distress in terms of depression, somatization, and anxiety. At both assessment points, the group that experienced lower initial exposure but then received less post-disaster help reported poorer QOL and psychological wellbeing. The two victim groups also differed significantly in changing trend along time. The group that received more support showed a general improvement in post-disaster wellbeing from three months to nine months.

Wang, Zhang, & Naotaka (1999) studied the quality of life in a rural community affected by a 6.2 degree earthquake in Hebei province, China, which occurred on January 10, 1998. Human Ss were 136 male and female Chinese adults (aged 18–60 yrs). Average education was 4.08 years. They lived in a village 0.5 miles from epicenter (Group A). A second group consisted of 199 male and female Chinese adults (aged 18–60 yrs). Average education was 4.42 years. They lived in a village 10 miles from the epicenter (Group B). A control group consisted of 172 male and female Chinese adults (mean age: 39.84 yrs) from a village unaffected by the earthquake. Ss were investigated three months after the earthquake by using 5-point scales in individual and family-member interviews. Data of Ss' earthquake suffering and experiences (death of family members or friends, injury, and money or property loss, pressure, support, and worries), psychological symptomatic distress, and quality of life (physical and mental well-being, mentality, social relationship, and environment) were compared. The results show that the village with a higher level of initial exposure to the earthquake and a higher level of post-earthquake support had a lower frequency of PTSD than the village with a lower level of initial exposure and less post-earthquake support. The rate of onset of DSM-IV PTSD within nine months for the two villages was 19.8% and 30.3%, respectively. In both villages, the rate of onset of earthquake-related PTSD within nine months was 24.2% by using DSM-IV criteria and 41.4% by using DSM-III-R criteria.

The use of the diagnosis of post traumatic stress disorder (PTSD) has not been very useful across cultures as it is based on the western cultural discourse that stress is an outcome of loss of control over nature. Priya (2002) provides a glimpse of suffering and healing among the survivors of an earthquake that occurred in 2001. An ethnographic approach was used for this study. It was found that the faith of the people that discharging their duties (karma) would lead them to peace and harmony with nature has resulted in better healing among the survivors in rural areas than among those in urban areas, where life is guided mainly by the materialistic goals. It is proposed that suffering and healing help to understand earthquake survivors better than PTSD.

Technological Disasters

Webb (1989) describes the accidental introduction of the fire retardant polybrominated biphenyl (PBB) into the food chain of Michigan in 1973 as an example of an insidious, slowly developing, and continuing technological catastrophe. D. M. Hartsough's (1985) transactional model of natural disasters was utilized to provide a conceptual framework for the psychological effects of the PBB crisis. Following this model, the event (toxic chemicals within the food chain) led to the quarantine of 576 farms, destruction of millions of animals and dairy products, and losses of $100-200 million. In spite of a high prevalence of depressive symptoms and somatic complaints, research results regarding psychological and physical effects of PBB poisoning have been equivocal and, at times, contradictory.

Hartsough's model points to possible intervention points that may have improved the response to the event and yielded fewer negative outcomes for the victims.

Tornadoes and Cyclonic (Hurricane) Disasters

Madakasira & O'Brien (1987) surveyed the mental health status of 116 disaster victims (aged 18–89 yrs) five months after a tornado devastated a rural community, using the Hopkins Symptom Checklist (HSCL) expanded to include most of the Diagnostic and Statistical Manual of Mental Disorders (DSM-III) criteria for posttraumatic stress disorder (PTSD). 69 Ss met the criteria for acute PTSD, 19 of whom had a severe form. Although an inadequate degree of social support was more often noted in victims with severe PTSD, other demographic factors and degree of injury or property damage did not appear to be related to the presence of PTSD. Severity or presence of PTSD was supported by high scores on all HSCL subscale factors. Findings suggest a high incidence of acute PTSD in victims of natural disasters and the potential value of HSCL in screening for PTSD in large populations.

Patrick & Patrick (1981) conducted a longitudinal study of psychological disturbance in 667 persons from 10 villages in Sri Lanka after the cyclone disaster of 1978. The post-cyclonic stress identified among the rural communities after their return to the same destroyed environment was studied. Symptoms (e.g., anxiety and suicidal ideation) tended to be early or delayed in appearance, and the degree of unpreparedness is postulated as the cause of the former.

Impact of Disasters in Rural Areas

The impact of disasters occurs in several major phases:

- Pre-impact (knowledge of legislation, resources, services)
- Immediate post-impact (information, coordination, crisis intervention techniques)
- Recovery (ongoing needs assessment)

Older people cope better and have strong stable relationships with a reserve of emotional experience. Children involved in disasters need special attention depending on age. If they have lost a family member, this is especially important. It is also important to pay attention to staff in the immediate post-impact phase when burnout is common.

PTSD is often looked at in relation to disasters at various levels. Shore, Vollmer, & Tatum (1989) analyzed lifetime rates for posttraumatic stress disorder (PTSD) in two rural Northwest US communities, one of which was affected by a major natural disaster, the eruption of Mount St. Helens. Individuals from the affected community were divided into groups of 410 low-exposure and 138 high-exposure Ss; 477 Ss from the other community served as controls. Community-wide rates of PTSD related to the disaster and to other events (e.g., combat, sexual assault) were identified. The community lifetime rate of PTSD was about 3% when measured by the Diagnostic and Statistical Manual of Mental Disorders (DSM-III). A much higher rate of disaster stress response syndromes was obtained for disaster victims when a broader definition including generalized anxiety disorder and depression was used.

The people living in the affected area will be experienced as a progression through the following phases:

Phases of Disaster

- Warning or Threat Phase
- Impact Phase
- Rescue or Heroic Phase
- Remedy or Honeymoon Phase
- Inventory Phase
- Disillusionment Phase
- Recovery Phase

Initial Impact

How, when, and where to proceed in responding to the disaster are questions that can only be answered for each disaster individually. While effective statewide planning can reduce and shorten this stage, some confusion and disorganization are inevitable during the early response. Experience is useful, but may not be readily adaptable to the current disaster. What if the State disaster coordinator is not available? Is there anyone else who knows what to do? Is anyone else within the State aware that funding for disaster crisis counseling is a possibility? Do local community mental health providers have their own plan for dealing with a disaster in their area? Do they know about the Stafford Act? Proper planning and experienced staff will minimize and shorten the period of confusion. Areas within the State where there is a higher level of disaster response organization and more frequent disasters may initiate response with less confusion.

Rural areas often find it more difficult to plan and mobilize for disaster preparedness and training for response. Confusion and disorientation can be minimized through statewide disaster planning and identification of a cadre of disaster response experts, nationally and statewide, who are willing to assist the State when requested. Even if preplanning has not occurred, early phases of a crisis counseling project can be less chaotic if the program staff has solid direction. In rural areas, there are a number of organizations that are already stakeholders in the wellbeing of the population in disaster. These groups will often begin providing services of various types immediately. Crisis counseling staff at this phase needs to be identifying and connecting with existing organizations. Contacting churches, unions, university extension services, fire or police auxiliaries, sheriff's departments, agricultural networks, civic groups like the Lions, Farm Bureau, Rotary, Optimists, Masons, and literally every group with concerns in the area can help in developing the needs assessment and a strategy for service delivery. Insurance agents and adjusters may also be good contacts. Even if a person's property is insured, they may still benefit from crisis counseling services in dealing with psychological recovery.

Phases of Rural Crisis Counseling

Despite the differences between the types of major disasters and geographic areas, the aftermath follows predictable phases. The disaster's impact on the physical, emotional, and spiritual health of the people living in the affected area will be experienced as a progression through the following phases: warning or threat, impact, rescue or heroic, remedy or honeymoon, inventory, disillusionment, and recovery (NIMH, 1983).

Phases of Disaster Recovery

Phase	Time Frame of Phase	Emotions	Behaviors	Most Important Resources
Heroic	Occurs at the time of impact and immediately afterward	Altruism. All emotions are strong and direct at this time.	Use of energy to save their own and others' lives and property.	Family groups, neighbors, and emergency teams
Honeymoon	From 1 week to 3 to 6 months after the disaster.	Strong sense of having shared a catastrophe experience and lived through it. Expectations of great assistance from official and government resources.	Victims clear out debris and wreckage, buoyed by promise of great help in rebuilding their lives.	Pre-existing community groups and emergent community groups which develop from specific needs caused by disaster.
Disillusionment	Lasts from 2 months to 1 or even 2 years.	Strong sense of disappointment, anger, resentment and bitterness appear if there are delays, failures, or unfulfilled hopes or promises of aid.	People concentrate on rebuilding their own lives and solving individual problems. The feeling of "shared community" is lost.	Many outside agencies may now pull out. Indigenous community agencies may weaken. Alternative resources may need to be explored.
Reconstruction	Lasts for several years following the disaster.	Victims realize that they need to solve the problem of rebuilding their lives. Visible recovery efforts serve to reaffirm the belief in themselves and the community. If recovery efforts are delayed, emotional problems which appear may be serious and intense.	People have assumed the responsibility for their own recovery. New construction programs and plans reaffirm the belief in capabilities and ability to recover.	Community groups with a long-term investment in the community and its people become key elements in this phase.

Phases often overlap; rather than being a discrete process, each phase blends with the others and will vary in response to the aspect of the disaster with which one is dealing at that moment. For example, a feeling of great pride and accomplishment (honeymoon phase) regarding the rescue of a family from flood waters may suddenly turn to anger or self-doubt (disillusionment phase) when one is reminded of another instance that ended in death.

The distress of dealing with a disaster depends upon an individual's interpretation of the event. The meaning assigned to a certain aspect of the disaster either helps or hinders the recovery process. Each individual responds and reacts from their own unique perceptions. The phases outlined here offer a predictable sequence of the human experience to disaster. Individuals experience distress differently. Predisposing factors, ambient stressors, physical health, community reactions, and actual and perceived levels of support influence the distress one experiences during and following the disaster. In the early phases of a disaster, the scope and intensity of their loss overwhelms most people. Commonly, in rural areas, the primary economic base is dependent upon natural resources. The immediate losses from any disaster are compounded in rural areas as the resources for continued existence are destroyed. The lands, lakes, fisheries, and enterprises that encompass the rural culture are more than a job. They form the economic base, value systems, and way of life for rural America.

Along with resources, rural residents often lose hope for the future. The recovery process must focus on the meaning of the disaster in a way that transforms the interpretation of being a helpless victim to one of being a successful survivor. Given the confusing maelstrom of need and emotion involved throughout the phases of disaster, the most important facets of the psychological healing process are validation and perspective. Disaster survivors/victims must hear that the reactions they are experiencing are normal and expected. They must also have access to discussions revolving around a realistic appraisal of the challenges presented and their options and response to those challenges. The crisis counseling project or disaster mental health professional may be the first source of perspective afforded a disaster survivor/victim.

Physical, social, emotional, and spiritual recovery takes place simultaneously but at different rates. An individual may be well into recovery physically, but still be distressed socially or emotionally. Given these realities, it is best to view disaster crisis counseling as assisting persons with a process of coping rather than seeing them through to some predetermined outcome. Crisis counseling services must be delivered in a way that provides connections to ongoing community services, such as social services, mental health providers, jobs and training programs, educational opportunities, financial services, and other services. In this way, the crisis counseling project equips disaster survivors with the capability of continuing their recovery as the phases progress (CMHS, 1994).

The key word in disaster circumstances is *change*. The massive changes in personal and community life cause physical, emotional, and social problems. Because these changes are dynamic and on-going, any program striving to be responsive to them must also be dynamic as well as flexible. When stress originates externally, *internal changes* occur. This is why certain events can cause a strong emotional reaction in one person and leave another indifferent. There are a number of factors that contribute to how one reacts to an event. These include the following:

Rescue or Heroic Phase

The Heroic Phase lasts from impact or pre-impact to approximately one week post-impact (this will be longer with more severe widespread events, e.g., Hurricane Katrina, Gulf oil spill, flooding in rural Pakistan). People respond to the demands of the situation by performing heroic acts to save lives and property. There is a sense of sharing with others who have been through the same experience. There is almost a feeling of "family", even with strangers. There is immediate support from family members both in and out of the area and by agency and governmental disaster personnel promising assistance. Feelings of euphoria are common. There is strong media support for the plight of the victims and the needs of the community. Activity levels are high. However, efficiency levels are low. Pain and loss, including physical pain, may not be recognized.

The most important resources during the Heroic Phase are family, neighbors, and emergency service responders. During the immediate post-impact phases, responders react and respond with high levels of energy, and seek information and facts. They develop and coordinate plans, equipment, and staff resources. Following the impact, adrenaline levels are high. Responders continue to push themselves through the stress signals and past warnings.

Honeymoon Phase

The Honeymoon Phase follows the Heroic Phase and may last for several weeks following the disaster. In the early parts of this phase, many survivors, even those who have sustained major losses, are feeling a sense of wellbeing for having survived. Shelters or schools may at first be seen as central meeting places to talk about shared experiences. They are also seen as being a safe place to stay until the survivors can return to their homes. Supported and encouraged by the promises of assistance by disaster relief personnel from voluntary and federal agencies, survivors clear the dirt and debris from their homes in anticipation of the help they believe will restore their lives.

The community as a whole pulls together in initial clean-up and distribution of supplies. In rural communities, neighbors often respond by pulling together and sharing resources with each other. Church and civic groups become active in meeting the various needs of the community. "Super Volunteers", who are not ready to deal with their own losses, work from dawn until after dark, helping their friends and neighbors get back on their feet. In the early parts of this stage, the community's expectations are extremely high. Their faith in those organizations' ability to help them recover is frequently unrealistic.

Some of the common emotional reactions during this stage include: adrenaline rush, anxiety, anger and frustration, survival guilt, restlessness, workaholism, risk-taking behaviors, and hyperactivity.

Disaster mental health professionals can assist during this stage by educating about common stress reactions and coping techniques, working with distressed clients, advocating for breaks and time off, defusing workers, team building, etc.

Disillusionment Phase

The greatest amount of frustration in the recovery process happens during the time it takes to process relief forms. The disaster event may be three or more weeks in the past before a disaster declaration is made. This time can be called a "Second Disaster". It is usually the period when the greatest amount of stress is seen because continual stressors are added to those experienced in the initial event. Victims must be encouraged to ventilate their built-up emotional energy.

The Disillusionment Phase lasts from one month to one or even two or more years. As the Honeymoon Phase passes into the Disillusionment Phase, the excitement of the media attention in the earlier phases begins to wane. Rather than feeling supported by the media, victims begin to feel that they are objects of insensitive curiosity. At the same time, they feel let down and isolated when the media no longer covers the story and moves on to other, fresher news. The departure of the media at the same time as victims are beginning to dig out can be extremely upsetting.

Victims begin to ask for answers, especially if the disaster could have been avoided, or if negligence of a person or agency was involved. Community support at this phase can be extremely important in determining the course of recovery.

During this phase, disaster mental health professionals work with clients, offer debriefings, defusings, and other crisis interventions for staff; mediate problems between staff and supervisors or clients; advocate for time off; educate about methods to decrease stress; and assist with team building as centers begin to consolidate and/or close down.

Reconstruction Phase

The final stage is the Reconstruction Phase. Victims come to the realization that the rebuilding of homes and businesses is primarily their responsibility. The rebuilding of the community reaffirms the victims' belief in themselves and the community. This phase may take from several years to the rest of their lives, depending on the amount of damage. If the rebuilding is delayed, the recovery process will also be delayed. Many of the disaster-related stress reactions will return when conditions are right for another disaster similar to the one the victims have experienced.

When the emergency response phase of the disaster is over, responders return to business as usual. They may experience frustration and loss after the intensity of the emergency situation. Local staff may also be victims, thus facing job pressures, as well as feeling overwhelmed by needs to complete their own recovery, feelings of loss, depression, anger, etc. By providing crisis intervention following a disaster, it is hoped that both responders and survivors can develop effective coping mechanisms that will assist them through the phases of recovery with less long-term emotional impact.

Stages often overlap. Rather than being a discrete process, each phase blends with the others and will vary in response to the aspect of the disaster with which one is dealing at that moment. For example, a feeling of great pride and accomplishment (honeymoon phase) regarding the rescue of a family from flood waters may suddenly turn to anger or self doubt (disillusionment phase) when one is reminded of another instance that ended in death. Much of the distress of dealing with a disaster depends upon one's interpretation of the event. The meaning one assigns to a certain aspect of the disaster either helps or hinders the recovery process. Individuals respond and react from their own unique point of view. Even though the phases outlined here offer a predictable sequence of the human experience in response to disaster. Predisposing factors, ambient stressors, physical health, community reactions, and actual and perceived levels of support influence the distress individuals experience during and following the impact. In early stages of a disaster, the scope and intensity of loss is overwhelming.

Commonly in rural areas, the primary economic base is dependent upon natural resources. The immediate losses from any disaster are compounded in rural areas as the resources for continued existence are destroyed. The lands, lakes, fisheries, and enterprises that encompass the rural culture are more than a job. They form the economic base, value systems, and way of life for rural America. Along with resources, rural residents often lose hope for the future. The recovery process must focus on the meaning of the disaster in a way that transforms the interpretation of being a helpless victim to one of being a successful survivor. Given the confusing maelstrom of need and emotion involved throughout the phases of disaster, the most important facets of the psychological healing process are validation and perspective. Disaster survivors/victims must hear that the reactions they are experiencing are normal and expected. They must also have access to discussions revolving around a realistic appraisal of the challenges presented and their options and response to those challenges. The crisis counseling program or disaster mental health responder may be the first source of perspective afforded a disaster survivor/victim.

Physical, social, emotional, and spiritual recovery takes place simultaneously but at different rates. An individual may be well into recovery physically, but still be distressed socially or emotionally. Given these realities, it is best to view disaster crisis counseling as assisting persons with a process of coping rather than seeing them through to some predetermined outcome.

Crisis counseling services must be delivered in a way that provides connections to ongoing community services, such as social services, mental health providers, jobs and training programs, educational opportunities, financial services, and other services. In this way, the crisis counseling project equips disaster survivors with the capability of continuing their recovery as the phases progress (CMHS, 1994). Massive changes in personal and community life cause physical, emotional, and social problems. These changes are dynamic and ongoing. Programs striving to be responsive to them must also be dynamic and flexible.

Crisis Counseling Programs are designed to last just short of a calendar year. Distinct stages of crisis counseling services can be tracked along with the phases of the disaster. The impact of these stages and their corresponding disaster phases on rural populations are described below:

Disaster Phases Affecting Rural Crisis Counseling

Despite the differences between types of major disasters and geographic areas, the aftermath follows predictable phases. The disaster's impact on the physical, emotional, and spiritual health of the people living in the affected area will be experienced as a progression through the disaster phases. Often, phases overlap or even repeat. Each phase blends with the others and varies in response to which aspect of the disaster one is dealing at that moment. A feeling of great pride and accomplishment (honeymoon phase) regarding the rescue of a family from flood waters can suddenly turn to anger or self doubt (disillusionment phase) if another instance ends in death or another significant loss.

The distress of dealing with a disaster depends upon one's perception and interpretation of the event. The meaning one assigns to a certain aspect of the disaster can help or hinder the recovery process. Individuals respond and react from their own unique perspective. While the phases of disaster offer a predictable sequence, individuals experience distress differently. Predisposing factors, ambient stressors, physical health, community reactions, actual and perceived levels of support influence the distress experienced during and following the impact of the disaster. In early phases, the scope and intensity of losses overwhelm most people.

Commonly, in rural areas, the primary economic base is dependent upon natural resources. The immediate losses from any disaster are compounded in rural areas as the resources for continued existence are destroyed. The lands, lakes, fisheries, and enterprises that encompass the rural culture are more than a job. Along with resources, rural residents often lose hope for the future. The recovery process must focus on the meaning of the disaster in a way that transforms the interpretation of being a helpless victim to one of being a successful survivor. Given the confusing maelstrom of need and emotion involved throughout the phases of disaster, the most important facets of the psychological healing process are validation and perspective. Responses, feelings, reactions, social, emotional and spiritual recovery questions are normal responses to an abnormal event. They often occur at different rates than physical recovery. Massive changes in personal and community life cause physical, emotional, and social problems. Changes are dynamic and ongoing. Programs also need to be dynamic and flexible.

Impact and Rescue or Heroic Phase

How, when, and where to proceed in responding to the disaster are questions that can only be answered for each disaster individually. While effective statewide planning can reduce and shorten this stage, during the early response some confusion and disorganization are inevitable. Experience is useful, but may not be readily adaptable to the current disaster. What if the State disaster coordinator is not available? Is there anyone else who knows what to do? Is anyone else within the State aware that funding for disaster crisis counseling is a possibility? Do local community mental health providers have their own plan for dealing with a disaster in their area? Do they know about the Stafford Act? Proper planning and experienced staff will minimize and shorten the period of confusion. Areas within the State where there is a higher level of disaster response organization and more frequent disasters may initiate response with less confusion.

Rural areas often find it more difficult to plan and mobilize for disaster preparedness and training for response. Confusion and disorientation can be minimized through statewide disaster planning and identification of a cadre of disaster response experts, nationally and statewide, who are willing to assist the State when requested.

Even without any preplanning, the early stages of the crisis counseling project can be less chaotic if the program staff has solid direction and goals. In rural areas, there are a number of organizations that are already stakeholders in the wellbeing of the population in disaster. These groups will often begin providing services of various types immediately. Crisis counseling staff at this stage needs to be identifying and connecting with existing organizations. Contacting churches, unions, university extension services, fire or police auxiliaries, sheriff's departments, agricultural networks, civic groups like the Lions, Farm Bureau, Rotary, Optimists, Masons and literally every group or concern in the area can help in developing the needs assessment and a strategy for service delivery. Insurance agents and adjusters may also be good contacts. Even if a person's property is insured, they may still benefit from crisis counseling services in dealing with psychological recovery.

Cultural Factors

Socio-demographic and cultural factors have been reported to shape help-seeking behavior. However, not much effort has been made to determine the effects of these factors on help-seeking among rural populations. Aderibigbe, Bloch, & Pandurangi (2003) employed a telephone survey using random-digit dialing to explore socio-demographic characteristics and ethnic differences in the types of professionals sought for unexplained somatic and emotional problems (N=1161) in rural eastern North Carolina. Ethnic differences in comfort with participating in support groups were also examined. The effect of a large natural disaster, Hurricane Floyd and subsequent flooding, on help-seeking choices and comfort with support groups was also assessed. Results suggested that the rural population makes a sharp distinction between somatic symptoms and stress-related symptoms. This distinction seemed more pronounced for European-Americans than for African-Americans. In general, African-Americans selected help-seeking from clergy more often than European-Americans, although for unexplained somatic symptoms, this difference was fostered by Hurricane Floyd with its flooding. African-Americans showed markedly increased comfort with support groups after the hurricane, while European-Americans showed no changes in comfort with support groups.

Sharan, Chaudhary, & Kavathekar (1996) examined psychiatric morbidity after a natural disaster in rural India. Semi-structured interviews were used to gather information from 56 individuals older than 14 yrs from 23 households in three villages affected by an earthquake. Diagnoses based on Diagnostic and Statistical Manual of Mental Disorders-III-Revised (DSM-III-R) criteria were assigned on the basis of the interviews, and nonparametric tests were applied to comparisons of Ss who were or were not given a psychiatric diagnosis. 33 Ss (59%) received a psychiatric diagnosis. The most common diagnoses were posttraumatic stress disorder (PTSD) (13 Ss) and major depression (12 Ss). Psychiatric morbidity was associated with female sex, and destruction of house and possessions. The mental health needs of disaster survivors in third world countries is indicated as an area needing further attention.

Crighton, Elliott & van der Meer (2003) researched the contribution of an environmental disaster to the psychosocial health of people living in Karakalpakstan, a semi-autonomous Republic in Uzbekistan. An interview survey was carried out by Medecins Sans Frontieres, with the assistance of the McMaster Institute of Environment and Health, local Universities, and local healthcare workers, on a random sample of 1118 individuals aged 18 years and older in three communities in Karakalpakstan in May/June 1999. The communities were chosen according to distance from the former seashore, urban/rural characteristics, and ethnic composition. The survey included questions about perceived general health, the General Health Questionnaire, the somatic symptom checklist of the Symptom Check List-90, questions about perceptions of the environmental disaster, social support as well as socio-demographic and socioeconomic characteristics. Findings show that 41% of all respondents reported environmental concern while 48% reported levels of somatic symptoms (SCL-90) associated with emotional distress above the normalized cut-point. Significant differences in levels of emotional distress were reported between men and women as well as between ethnic groups.

Hutton (2003) examined the impact of riverine hazards and displacement upon displaced persons, both males and females, in Bangladesh. The specific objectives of the study were to:

- Determine the magnitude of psychological distress associated with riverine hazards and displacement in Bangladesh

- Examine patterns and predictors related to the economic, social, and psychological adaptation of male and female displaced persons

- Identify patterns of psychological coping common to displaced persons

Research was conducted during the 1998 flood season in Bangladesh. Subjects consisted of 238 displaced persons randomly sampled from four squatter settlements in the city of Serajganj in Bangladesh. A comparison group of 223 demographically comparative non-displaced persons was drawn from three rural villages in the thana (sub-district) of Shariakandi. Structured interviews were conducted at the respondents' households over a six week period using trained university students. The findings show that the constant threat of riverbank erosion has contributed to the development of a distinct set of characteristics related to disaster-induced displacement in Bangladesh. Although frequent displacement is common among the floodplain residents, less than one-fifth of the displaced persons had perceived riverbank erosion to be a serious problem and just one-tenth believed they would eventually be permanently displaced.

Although they exhibited significantly higher level of distress than the non-displaced, this was related primarily to socioeconomic deprivation rather than displacement per se. The commonly hypothesized factors such as loss of land and frequency and duration of displacement were not found to have a significant association with distress levels. Among both displaced and non-displaced, chronic survival concerns, daily hunger, and marginal living conditions were predictive factors of psychological distress. The need to integrate disaster management within a social, cultural, and psychological context was emphasized. Popular development and psychological theory usually associate low personal control with maladaptive passivity and dependency. In this study, displaced persons more often responded to their difficulties with active problem-solving efforts, with fatalism being among the least utilized forms of coping. It appears that low aspirations and self-efficacy generated by poverty may in some instances be psychologically adaptive. These attributes can reduce levels of frustration and distress, without diminishing determination and perseverance.

McDowell (2002) notes that research on impoverishment risks arising out of development-induced, involuntary population displacement is improving the understanding of rural development processes more generally. Following comparative studies of the process of livelihood destruction and re-establishment dynamics among communities resettled as a result of planned development and war, McDowell develops a methodological framework for post-disaster reconstruction research. He outlines a research methodology to conduct and organize theory-led fieldwork on the socio-economic and cultural impacts of forced population displacement, involuntary resettlement, and livelihood reconstruction. Combining recent Sustainable Livelihoods research and the concept of Impoverishment Risks and Reconstruction, McDowell suggests that a focus on institutions and sustainability will help shape research to better understand the impacts of disasters and induced-displacement processes on the livelihoods of affected populations.

Conclusions and Approaches

Psychologists and other mental health professionals are encouraged to broaden their skills to include training in disaster intervention as global awareness of the need for disaster mental health increases. As members of the Association of Virgin Islands Psychologists, Dudley-Grant, Mendez, & Zinn (2000) recount their experiences as professionals and as individuals when violent hurricanes hit the U.S. Virgin Islands. They provide suggestions for individual and community-level interventions as well as potential collaborations with disaster relief agencies such as the American Red Cross and the Federal Emergency Management Agency. They discuss unique concerns related to working in multicultural settings, rural service delivery, and research opportunities.

Zargar, Najarian, & Roger (1993) focused on the association between psychological aspects of disasters and the process of reconstructing both dwellings and the community infrastructure. They took into account the existing literature on the subject as well as the results of survey data obtained from resettled rural survivors of the Iraq-Iran conflict. They suggest that two theoretical models are particularly relevant to disasters: life events and learned helplessness. It is important to review the factors affecting the implementation of reconstruction policies. This includes focusing on the provision of emergency and temporary shelter, examining factors which govern the timing of the return of the survivors to the new site and including consideration of the role of the survivors themselves during the reconstruction process (in relation to decision-making and physical rebuilding).

Silver & Goldstein (1992) introduced a model for the classification of crisis intervention and disaster services as being:

- clinic-based, ad hoc,
- school-oriented
- disaster service based
- integrative

An example is presented of an integrative-collaborative model that was developed to cope with situations of suicide, accidental death, or natural disaster, when they occur in rural areas and small towns. The Community Crisis Intervention Team (CCIT) was developed with characteristics specific to a collaborative model. This is somewhat similar to the CISM Teams set up in other communities.

Hessen (1989) discusses the psychosocial support provided by a psychiatric outpatient clinic at a small rural hospital in Norway in connection with a plane crash that produced 36 casualties. The disaster training of human service workers, psychiatric emergency plans, emotional support, cooperation between health and social services, long-term support functions, use of the media, responsibility for support work, use of experts on psychosocial intervention in crisis work, and work routines for and psychological debriefing of psychiatric personnel are considered.

The use of laptop computers for data gathering and resource searches has become very valuable as a tool in many settings in recent years. Adaptation to uses in disaster aftermaths and other crisis and critical incident situations is just beginning to become more common. Echterling & Hoschar (1989) describe the use of the personal computer in a rural mental health program designed to address disaster-induced psychological problems following a flood. The computer was used in the desktop publication of pamphlets for disaster survivors and for:

- Managing data to assess the needs of survivors
- Setting priorities
- Planning interventions
- Keeping records
- Generating reports

The computer also was used in mailing letters to survivors, providing them with updated information regarding available services and continuing concerns, and evaluating effectiveness.

Information about clergy responses to crises and disasters in rural areas is not very extensive, especially in areas of the rural American west. Echterling, Bradfield, & Wylie (1988) contrasted the roles, activities, and stresses of 24 urban and rural ministers in responding to the November 1985 flood in West Virginia and Virginia. Ss completed questionnaires, 7–26 months after the flood, that assessed the challenges they faced, the special contributions they offered survivors, and the problems they experienced in their disaster work. Urban and rural Ss faced similar challenges, such as helping people to integrate disasters into the theological context of their religious beliefs. However, they often differed in the resources available to them, in the variety of disaster relief roles they took, and in the strategies they pursued in ministering to the needs of their communities.

Southeast Wyoming Mental Health Center in Wyoming sponsored a workshop in crisis intervention as a means of training non-mental health professionals (mainly ministers) in abilities to deal more adequately with mental health problems (Oetting, Cole, & Adams, 1969). Several techniques frequently used in eliciting and recording proceedings were unacceptable to this group because of their professional orientation, so some aspects of the workshop were incomplete. It was concluded that participants need to know the worth of evaluation, that all staff participants should have a positive view about the project and be thoroughly familiar with the evaluation plan. This should include more than one kind of information gathering.

Different approaches following disasters in rural areas need to be tailored to the communities and groups affected. Heffron (1977) discusses Project Outreach, a specially designed crisis intervention program funded by the National Institute of Mental Health following the devastating 1972 Agnes flood disaster in the Wyoming

Valley of northeastern Pennsylvania. The project was in operation for 32 months and employed 60 individuals, primarily specially-trained, indigenous nonprofessionals. Utilizing a neighborhood canvassing effort, Human Service Counselors encountered individuals with a wide range of problems, varying in severity and difficulty from those requiring limited assistance from community resources to those involving the need for direct mental health services. Over 25,000 client contacts were made. The project demonstrated that a cadre of local residents can be recruited, selected, and trained within a very short period of time to provide crisis intervention services to disaster victims. Further, Project Outreach has shown that an active, community-based, outreach/case-finding effort can be a highly effective approach in dealing with the problems of disaster victims.

The National Institute of Mental Health (NIMH) has emphasized improved mental health and mental health services in rural areas through funding for research projects and research centers (Hutner & Windle, 1991). The five research areas include:

- The epidemiology of mental disorders
- Behavioral and psychological factors of mental illness and health
- Mental health services
- Community support demonstration programs
- Child and adolescent service system demonstration programs

NIMH has also supported related activities including:

- State planning
- Improvement of state data systems
- Protection of and advocacy for mentally ill individuals
- Disaster relief
- Professional training
- Education concerning depression

It is suggested that those planning work in these areas contact NIMH for current and up-to-date information.

Despite the differences between types of major disasters and geographic areas, the aftermath follows predictable phases. The disaster's impact on the physical, emotional, and spiritual health of people living in the affected area is experienced as a progression through the following phases: warning or threat, impact, rescue or heroic, remedy or honeymoon, inventory, disillusionment, and recovery (NIMH, 1983). Rural areas often find it more difficult to plan and mobilize for disaster preparedness and training for response. Confusion and disorientation can be minimized through statewide disaster planning and identification of a cadre of disaster response experts, nationally and statewide, who are willing to assist when requested.

Disaster Mental Health in Rural Environments

Rural Crisis Intervention

Mental health services before, during and following disasters, critical incidents, crises, and terrorist activities are becoming an integral part of disaster, crisis, and critical incident preparedness, mitigation, response, and follow-up (Provenzo & Fradd, 1995; Gist & Lubin, 1999). Disaster Mental Health Services (DMHS) is a relatively new field which has expanded significantly within the past 15 years (since Hurricane Andrew). Critical Incident Stress Management (CISM) and Critical Incident Stress Debriefing (CISD) have been around since the early 1980s (Mitchell & Everly, 1993).

Disasters in Rural Areas

Disasters occur everywhere. Preparation for their aftermath is more often accomplished in areas which are prone to certain types of disaster (e.g. hurricanes, floods, tornadoes). Planning for these in rural environments has improved over the years and responses by disaster agencies (e.g. FEMA) have helped. However, there are other forms of disaster and critical incidents that can and do occur in rural areas as well as urban ones (e.g. critical incidents such as shootings, vehicle accidents, house fires, acts of terrorism, hazmat spills, wildfires, hostage situations, spousal and child abuse, and others).

Resources for the aftermath of these are not as readily available nor as extensive as in more urban environments. Farberow (1985) discusses the mental health component of disaster relief, which was incorporated in Public Law 93-288 in the 1970s and mandated the National Institute of Mental Health to provide counseling services and training materials. The impact of disasters as outlined above, occurs in several major phases: pre-impact (knowledge of legislation, resources, services), immediate post-impact (information, coordination, crisis intervention techniques), and recovery (ongoing needs assessment). Special attention is needed for children involved in disasters, especially if they lose a family member, and for staff and first responders in the immediate post-impact phase when burnout is common.

McRee, Corder, & Deitz (1985–1986) outline the experiences of a voluntary intervention team that aided in providing mental health services to children in a tornado disaster area. Topics include administrative issues and services provided by the team. They suggest that this information may be helpful in planning and programming for other agencies involved in similar crisis interventions in rural communities.

Critical Incidents and Crisis Intervention

Critical incidents are, fortunately, not as common in rural as in urban areas. However, they do occur and do have significant impacts on communities, those directly involved, and on responders.

Silver & Goldstein (1992) suggested a model for the classification of crisis intervention and disaster services as being clinic-based, ad hoc, school-oriented, disaster service based, and integrative. An example is presented of an integrative-collaborative model that was developed to cope with situations of suicide, accidental death, or natural disaster when they occur in rural areas and small towns. The Community Crisis Intervention Team (CCIT) was developed with characteristics specific to a collaborative model. The distinctive qualities of the CCIT are identified and discussed within the context of a case study of an intervention in a school setting following an adolescent's suicide.

There is a good amount of literature that discusses the CISM/CISD process in various settings. This information can be used in rural settings as well.

Disaster and Crisis Impacts in Rural Areas

Crises

Conditions in the West and ranching culture, including the rural geography, the cowboy mystique, the social fabric of the rural lifestyle, and the "health" of agriculture can negatively impact the delivery of rural health services and the attitude of ranchers and farmers toward seeking help for personal problems. These conditions may create a behavioral hazard to ranchers, farmers, and individuals in the West. It is important to understand and develop strategies that exist to improve the availability and acceptance of rural behavioral health services. Emergency crews in rural areas face certain challenges that urban crews may not. These challenges center mainly around the fact that people in small communities tend to know each other and that many emergency workers are volunteers who give up time with their families to work in the service of their communities. Studies have shown that small rural communities require a different kind of attention because of their unique characteristics (Farberow, 1985). These include pride in independence, rejection of the unfamiliar, a tendency to take problems to family rather than professionals, a larger number of persons living well below the poverty line, and less acceptance of mental illness.

PTSD is often looked at in relation to disasters at various levels. Shore, Vollmer & Tatum (1989) analyzed lifetime rates for posttraumatic stress disorder (PTSD) in two rural Northwest US communities, one of which was affected by a major natural disaster, the eruption of Mount St Helens. Individuals from the affected community were divided into groups of 410 low-exposure and 138 high-exposure Ss; 477 Ss from the other community served as controls. Community-wide rates of PTSD related to the disaster and to other events (e.g., combat, sexual assault) were identified. The community lifetime rate of PTSD was about 3% when measured by the Diagnostic and Statistical Manual of Mental Disorders (DSM-III). A much higher rate of disaster stress response syndromes was obtained for disaster victims when a broader definition including generalized anxiety disorder and depression was used.

Rural Crisis Intervention

Mental health services before, during, and following disasters, critical incidents, crises, and terrorist activities are becoming an integral part of disaster, crisis and critical incident preparedness, mitigation, response, and follow-up (Provenzo & Fradd, 1995; Gist & Lubin, 1999). Disaster Mental Health Services (DMHS) is a relatively new field which has expanded significantly within the past 15 years (since Hurricane Andrew). Critical Incident Stress Management (CISM) and Critical Incident Stress Debriefing (CISD) have been around since the early 1980s (Mitchell & Everly, 1993).

Disasters In Rural Areas

Preparation for the aftermath of disasters is more often accomplished in areas which are prone to certain types of disaster (e.g. hurricanes, floods, tornadoes). While planning for disasters in rural environments has improved over the years and responses by disaster agencies (e.g. FEMA) have helped, there are other forms of disaster and critical incidents that can and do occur in rural areas as well as urban ones. These include critical incidents such as shootings, vehicle accidents, house fires, acts of terrorism, hazmat spills, wildfires, hostage situations, spousal and child abuse, and others).

McRee, Corder, & Deitz (1985-1986) outline the experiences of a voluntary intervention team that aided in providing mental health services to children in a tornado disaster area. Topics include administrative issues and services provided by the team. They suggest that this information may be helpful in planning and programming for other agencies involved in similar crises interventions in rural communities.

Critical Incidents and Crisis Intervention

Critical incidents are, fortunately, not as common in rural as in urban areas. However, they do occur and do have significant impacts on communities, those directly involved and on responders. Silver & Goldstein (1992) suggested a model for the classification of crisis intervention and disaster services as being clinic-based, ad hoc, school-oriented, disaster service based, and integrative. They present an example of an integrative-collaborative model which was developed to cope with situations of suicide, accidental death, or natural disaster when they occur in rural areas and small towns. Community Crisis Intervention Teams (CCIT) were developed using a collaborative model. The distinctive qualities of the CCIT were identified and discussed within the context of a case study involving an intervention in a school setting following an adolescent's suicide. There is a large amount of literature that discusses the CISM/CISD process in various settings. This information can be used in rural settings as well.

Additional Considerations

Families and Children

Earls, Smith & Reich (1988) report on a pilot study examining the reactions of children to a disaster of severe flooding in a circumscribed area of rural Missouri. Both parents and 6-17 yr old children (32 parent-child pairs) were interviewed separately approximately one year after the flood, using parallel versions of a structured diagnostic interview designed to identify children with Diagnostic and Statistical Manual of Mental Disorders (DSM-III) diagnoses. Results document the importance of interviewing children directly. Children reported more anxiety symptoms than parents reported for their children. Although symptoms of posttraumatic stress were reported, none of the children met full criteria for the disorder. Children most likely to be adversely affected were those with a pre-existing disorder and those with parents who also reported a high number of symptoms in themselves.

In another study of post-disaster effects on children, 32 mothers and their children (aged 6-17 yrs) who had been exposed to severe flooding in rural Mississippi were interviewed, using the Diagnostic Interview for Children and Adolescents. Other sources of information about the children included school reports and the teachers' version of the Child Behavior Checklist. Results indicate that in most cases of psychiatric disorder, the diagnosis could have been made from the child's report alone. Children as young as six years of age reported emotional problems of which the parent appeared unaware. The decision-making process used in the assignment of summary psychiatric diagnoses based on child and parent reports, as well as a number of other sources of information about the child are important factors to consider when doing assessments (Reich & Earls, 1987).

The farm crisis in the 1980's provided some insights into how rural families cope with crises. For example, data from 77 adolescents in farm and ranch families were used to examine the relationship of demographic variables, family stressor events, and family coping strategies to adolescent adaptation (Plunkett, Henry & Knaub, 1999). Results indicated that adolescent age and family transitions were positively related to individual stress. Males reported less family stress than did females. Seeking spiritual support was negatively related to family stress, while the perceived impact of the farm crisis was positively related to family stress. Family support was positively related, and family substance use issues were negatively related, to adolescent satisfaction with family life.

Hargrove (1986) suggested clinical and community activities for mental health workers during the farm crisis of the 1980's. He maintained that a model for understanding human response to natural disasters is useful for understanding responses to farm crises. He made recommendations for communities and suggested that the clinical/advocate model developed by G. B. Melton (1983; see also PA, Vol 61:9256) is a useful approach. Forrest (1988) suggests that the rural family, is vulnerable to overwhelming crises and such events can contribute to adolescent suicide. In a more positive direction, Thompson & McCubbin (1987) outline resource materials that are available to help educators, counselors, and others to support rural familes in crises and facilitate decision making, long-range planning, and problem solving. Counseling programs, workshops, publications, support groups for coping with stress, and computerized decision aids are among approaches discussed.

Some Steps in Helping Children Following Disaster

A basic principle in working with children who have experienced disaster is that they are essentially normal children who have experienced great stress. Most of the problems that appear are related to the disaster and are usually transitory in nature. The process suggested for assisting families and children most often begins with "crisis intervention". The primary goal in crisis intervention is to identify, respond to, and relieve the stresses that result from the crisis (disaster) and to re-establish normal functioning as quickly as possible. Sometimes this reaction is mild. However, at other times it can be severe. It is important that workers recognize when the condition is mild and can usually be handled by families with a little guidance. It is also important to recognize when referral to a professional is important, such as a school counselor or when the condition is severe and requires intervention by a mental health professional. Following are some suggested steps in this helping process:

1. Establish Rapport

- Let the children know that you are interested in them and want to help.
- Check with the children to make sure that they understand what you are
- saying and that *you* understand them.
- Display genuine respect and regard for the children and their families.
- Communicate trust and promise only that which you can do.
- Convey acceptance of the children and their families.
- Communicate to the children and their families that you are an informed authority.

2. Identify, Define, and Focus on the Problem

- Identify and prioritize specific problems with the children, parents and family.
- Select a specific problem, define its characteristics, and focus on solving it first.
- Achieve a quick resolution to the problem so that the members of the family experience a sense of success and control.
- Evaluate the seriousness of each of the identified problems and the capacity of the family to deal with them.

3. Understanding Feelings

- Demonstrate your ability to see and feel as others do.
- Display patience in trying to understand children's feelings as children are frequently unable to express their fears.

- Respond to children's stories often by commenting on the events and affirming their feelings.

- Express a nurturing positive regard for the children to help convey an appreciation for the kind and intensity of their feelings.

4. Listening Carefully

- Understand the disaster concerns from the point of view of the children.

- Listen to the children's account of the disaster many times in order to help children "work through" their feelings associated with the disaster.

- Refrain from interrupting the children as they tell their stories.

- Affirm children's feelings by giving them time to express themselves.

5. Communicating Clearly

- Communicate in a language children understand.

- Talk with children in groups or with siblings or other family members.

- Seek the presence of family members to help interpret "code words" used by the children.

- Communicate with children in their dominant language.

Role of the Family

The child's family can be defined in terms of the significant persons who provide care and support and who are also members of the child's nuclear and extended family structure. Because children usually live in family systems, both the experience of the disaster and the recovery from its aftermath are often mutually experienced. As a result, children will share common aspects of the disaster experience. Re-telling these experiences by the adults and the children in the family can help normalize the overwhelming rush of feelings associated with disaster. The role of the worker is usually to simply give the families permission to share their feelings with each other and to communicate that having disaster related feelings is normal and that sharing these feelings with each other is appropriate and healthy.

One of the functions of crisis counseling in disasters is psychoeducation to convey information to parents about the common reactions families have to trauma and loss following a disaster. Parents often deny the need for this type of information for themselves. However, they will gladly participate in programs or other gatherings where this type of information is provided for helping support their children. Parents will typically recognize stress reactions and accompanying behavioral changes in their children before recognizing them in themselves. Mental health workers help all members of the family unit by sensitizing parents to the signs of stress in their children and suggesting strategies for helping their children.

Workers can remind parents of the following suggestions:

- Parents should acknowledge the parts of the disaster that were frightening to them and other adults.

- Parents should not falsely minimize the danger as it will not end a child's concerns.

- The child's age affects how he or she will respond to the disaster. (e.g. a six year old may express his or her concerns by refusing to attend school, while an adolescent may express his or her concerns by arguing more with parents.).

- The way the child sees and understands his or her parent's response is very important.

- Parents should admit their concerns and also stress their abilities to cope with the situation.

Usually the family's role is simply to learn to work together in order to solve problems and to actively recognize the needs and feelings of both the children and the adults. The identification of concrete issues which are problematic for the family as well as for individuals within the family is usually the first step toward emotional recovery for the family. This should be followed by designing solutions to problems, resolving problems by implementing solutions, and recognizing the success of positively resolving problems. As such, family members can begin to re-establish a sense of mastery over their environment and bring equilibrium back to the roles of each family member. By continued use of this process during the phases of recovery, family members become closer as a family unit and individually more autonomous. This can help all family members to re-establish their identity and to continue with their normal developmental roles.

When working with families from diverse cultural and rural backgrounds, it is important for workers to be sensitive to language differences and cultural needs. Quite often children get thrust into the role of interpreter if their parents and relatives are not fluent in English. Such responsibility may require skills beyond the child's current stage of development and be too stressful for the child. The worker can relieve the child of this responsibility by seeking out adult interpreters for the family.

Some Common Feelings and Behaviors

One method of assessing signs and symptoms displayed following stressful events is to utilize the BASIC-ID outlined by Arnold Lazarus (1976, 1989, 2000). Some of the common reactions expressed by children include the following:

Behavior

- Avoiding reminders
- Crying easily
- Change in appetite
- Talking repeatedly about the event
- Refusal to go to school
- Repetitive play

Affect

- Depression or sadness
- Irritability, anger, resentfulness
- Despair, hopelessness, feelings of guilt
- Phobias, health concerns
- Anxiety or fearfulness

Somatic Complaints

- Exacerbation of medical problems
- Headaches
- Fatigue
- Physical complaints with no physical cause

Interpersonal Skills

- Arguments with family and friends
- Increased conflicts with family
- Social withdrawal

Cognitive

- Trouble concentrating
- Preoccupation with the event

- Questioning spiritual beliefs
- Inability to process the significance of the event

Imagery

- Intrusive thoughts
- Sleep problems
- Recurring dreams or nightmares

Drugs/Alcohol

- Use of drugs/alcohol to avoid problems

The above list is not all-inclusive and should be used only as a guide. It will need to be used with different emphases depending upon age and developmental levels.

Cultural Factors

Socio-demographic and cultural factors assist in developing help-seeking behavior. Aderibigbe, Bloch & Pandurangi (2003) employed a telephone survey using random-digit dialing to explore socio-demographic characteristics and ethnic differences in the types of professionals sought for unexplained somatic and emotional problems (N=1161) in rural eastern North Carolina. Ethnic differences in comfort with participating in support groups were also examined. The effect of a large natural disaster (Hurricane Floyd and subsequent flooding) on help-seeking choices and comfort with support groups was also assessed. Results suggested that rural populations make a sharp distinction between somatic symptoms and stress-related symptoms. This distinction seemed more pronounced among European-Americans than African-Americans. In general, African-Americans selected help-seeking from clergy more often than European-Americans. For unexplained somatic symptoms this difference was fostered by Hurricane Floyd with its flooding. African-Americans showed markedly increased comfort with support groups after the hurricane, while European-Americans showed no changes in comfort with support groups.

Sharan, Chaudhary & Kavathekar (1996) examined psychiatric morbidity after a natural disaster in rural India. Semi-structured interviews were used to gather information from 56 individuals older than 14 yrs from 23 households in three villages affected by an earthquake. Diagnoses based on Diagnostic and Statistical Manual of Mental Disorders-III-Revised (DSM-III-R) criteria were assigned on the basis of the interviews, and nonparametric tests were applied to comparisons of Ss who were or were not given a psychiatric diagnosis. 33 Ss (59%) received a psychiatric diagnosis. The most common diagnoses were posttraumatic stress disorder (PTSD) (13 Ss) and major depression (12 Ss). Psychiatric morbidity was associated with female sex, and destruction of house and possessions. The mental health needs of disaster survivors in third world countries is indicated as an area needing further attention

Crighton, Elliott & van der Meer (2003) researched the contribution of an environmental disaster to the psychosocial health of people living in Karakalpakstan, a semi-autonomous Republic in Uzbekistan. An interview survey was carried out by Medecins Sans Frontieres, with the assistance of the McMaster Institute of Environment and Health, local Universities and local health care workers, on a random sample of 1118 individuals aged 18 years and older in three communities in Karakalpakstan in May/June 1999. The communities were chosen according to distance from the former seashore, urban/rural characteristics and ethnic composition. The survey included questions about perceived general health, the General Health Questionnaire, the somatic symptom checklist of the Symptom Check List-90, questions about perceptions of the environmental disaster, social support as well as sociodemographic and socioeconomic characteristics. Findings show that 41% of all respondents reported environmental concern while 48% reported levels of somatic symptoms (SCL-90) associated with emotional distress, above the normalized cut-point. Significant differences in levels of emotional distress were reported between men and women as well as between ethnic groups.

Hutton (2003) examined the impact of riverine hazards and displacement upon displaced persons, both males and females, in Bangladesh. The specific objectives of the study were to:

- Determine the magnitude of psychological distress associated with riverine hazards and displacement in Bangladesh,

- Examine patterns and predictors related to the economic, social, and psychological adaptation of male and female displaced persons, and

- Identify patterns of psychological coping common to displaced persons.

Research was conducted during the 1998 flood season in Bangladesh. Subjects consisted of 238 displaced persons randomly sampled from four squatter settlements in the city of Serajganj in Bangladesh. A comparison group of 223 demographically comparative non-displaced persons was drawn from three rural villages in the thana (sub-district) of Shariakandi. Structured interviews were conducted at the respondents' households over a six week period using trained university students. The findings show that the constant threat of riverbank erosion has contributed to the development of a distinct set of characteristics related to disaster-induced displacement in Bangladesh. Although frequent displacement is common among the floodplain residents, less than one-fifth of the displaced persons had perceived riverbank erosion to be a serious problem and just one-tenth believed they would eventually be permanently displaced. Although they exhibited significantly higher level of distress than non-displaced, this was related primarily to socioeconomic deprivation rather than displacement per se. The commonly hypothesized factors such as loss of land and frequency and duration of displacement were not found to have a significant association with distress levels. Among both displaced and non-displaced, chronic survival concerns, daily hunger, and marginal living conditions were predictive factors of psychological distress. The need to integrate disaster management within a social, cultural and psychological context was emphasized. Popular development and psychological theory usually associates low personal control with maladaptive passivity and dependency. In this study, displaced persons more often responded to their difficulties with active problem-solving efforts, with fatalism being among the least utilized forms of coping. It appears that low aspirations and self-efficacy generated by poverty may in some instances be psychologically adaptive. These attributes can reduce levels of frustration and distress, without diminishing determination and perseverance.

McDowell (2002) notes that research on impoverishment risks arising out of development-induced involuntary population displacement is improving the understanding of rural development processes more generally. Following comparative studies of the process of livelihood destruction and re-establishment dynamics among communities resettled as a result of planned development and war, McDowell develops a methodological framework for post-disaster reconstruction research. He outlines a research methodology to conduct and organize theory-led fieldwork on the socio-economic and cultural impacts of forced population displacement, involuntary resettlement, and livelihood reconstruction. Combining recent Sustainable Livelihoods research and the concept of Impoverishment Risks and Reconstruction, McDowell suggests that a focus on institutions and sustainability will help shape research to better understand the impacts of disasters and induced-displacement processes on the livelihoods of affected populations.

Conclusions and Approaches

Psychologists and other mental health professionals are encouraged to broaden their skills to include training in disaster intervention as global awareness of the need for disaster mental health increases. As members of the Association of Virgin Islands Psychologists, Dudley-Grant, Mendez & Zinn (2000) recount their experiences as professionals and as individuals when violent hurricanes hit the U.S. Virgin Islands. They provide suggestions for individual and community-level interventions as well as potential collaborations with disaster relief agencies such as the American Red Cross and the Federal Emergency Management Agency. They discuss unique concerns related to working in multicultural settings, rural service delivery, and research opportunities.

Zargar, Najarian & Roger (1993) focused on the association between psychological aspects of disasters and the process of reconstructing both dwellings and the community infrastructure. They took into account the existing literature on the subject as well as the results of survey data obtained from resettled rural survivors of the Iraq-Iran conflict. They suggest that two theoretical models are particularly relevant to disasters: life events and learned helplessness. It is important to review the factors affecting the implementation of reconstruction policies. This includes focusing on the provision of emergency and temporary shelter, examining factors which govern the timing of the return of the survivors to the new site and including consideration of the role of the survivors themselves during the reconstruction process (in relation to decision-making and to physical rebuilding).

Silver & Goldstein (1992) introduced a model for the classification of crisis intervention and disaster services as being:

- Clinic-based, ad hoc
- School-oriented
- Disaster service based
- Integrative

An example is presented of an integrative-collaborative model that was developed to cope with situations of suicide, accidental death, or natural disaster when they occur in rural areas and small towns. The Community Crisis Intervention Team (CCIT) was developed with characteristics specific to a collaborative model. This is somewhat similar to the CISM Teams set up in other communities.

Hessen (1989) discusses the psychosocial support provided by a psychiatric outpatient clinic at a small rural hospital in Norway in connection with a plane crash that produced 36 casualties. The disaster training of human service workers, psychiatric emergency plans, emotional support, cooperation between health and social services, long-term support functions, use of the media, responsibility for support work, use of experts on psychosocial intervention in crisis work, and work routines for and psychological debriefing of psychiatric personnel are considered.

The use of laptop computers for data gathering and resource searches has become very valuable as a tool in many settings in recent years. Adaptation to uses in disaster aftermaths and other crisis and critical incident situations is just beginning to become more common. Echterling & Hoschar (1989) describe the use of the personal computer in a rural mental health program designed to address disaster-induced psychological problems following a flood. The computer was used in the desktop publication of pamphlets for:

- Disaster survivors
- Managing data to assess the needs of survivors
- Setting priorities
- Planning interventions
- Keeping records
- Generating reports

The computer also was used in mailing letters to survivors, providing them with updated information regarding available services and continuing concerns, and evaluating effectiveness.

Information about clergy responses to crises and disasters in rural areas is not very extensive, especially in areas of the rural American west. Echterling, Bradfield & Wylie (1988) contrasted the roles, activities, and stresses of 24 urban and rural ministers in responding to the November 1985 flood in West Virginia and Virginia. Ss completed questionnaires 7-26 months after the flood that assessed the challenges they faced, the special contributions they offered survivors, and the problems they experienced in their disaster work. Urban and rural Ss faced similar challenges, such as helping people to integrate disasters into the theological context of their religious beliefs. However, they often differed in the resources available to them, in the variety of disaster relief roles they took, and in the strategies they pursued in ministering to the needs of their communities.

The National Institute of Mental Health (NIMH) has emphasized improved mental health and mental health services in rural areas through funding for research projects and research centers (Hutner & Windle (1991). The five research areas include:

NIMH has also supported related activities including:

- The epidemiology of mental disorders

- Behavioral and psychological factors of mental illness and health

- Health mental services

- Community support demonstration programs

- Child and adolescent service system demonstration programs

- State planning

- Improvement of state data systems

- Protection of and advocacy for mentally ill individuals

- Disaster relief

- Professional training

- Education concerning depression

It is suggested that those planning work in these areas contact NIMH for more current and up-to-date information.

Perception of the Event

- **When the event is perceived realistically:** There is an awareness of the relationship between the event and the sensations of stress, which in itself will reduce the tension. It is likely that the state of stress will be resolved effectively.

- **When the perception of the event is distorted:** There is no awareness of the connection between the event and the feeling of stress. Any attempt to resolve the problem will be affected accordingly.

- **Hypotheses to verify** concerning the individual's perception of the event:
    o   What meaning does the event have in the person's eyes?
    o   How will it affect his/her future?
    o   Is he/she able to look at it realistically? Or does he/she misinterpret its meaning?

Support by the Natural Network

Support by the natural network means the support given by people in the individual's immediate circle who are accessible and who can be relied on to help at that time. In a stressful situation, the lack or inadequacy of resources can leave an individual in a vulnerable position conducive to a state of disequilibrium or crisis.

Mechanisms of Adaptation

These mechanisms reduce the tension and help promote adaptation to stressful situations. They can be activated consciously or unconsciously. Throughout life, individuals learn to use various methods to adapt to anxiety and reduce tension. These mechanisms aim at maintaining and protecting their equilibrium. When an event happens which causes stress, and the learned mechanisms of adaptation are not effective, the discomfort is experienced at a conscious level.

Returning to Equilibrium

Mental health is described by Antoine Parot as "a psychic ability to function in a harmonious, agreeable, effective manner, when circumstances allow, to cope flexibly with difficult situations and to re-establish one's dynamic equilibrium after a test."

Every time a stressful event happens, there are certain recognized compensating factors which can help promote a return to equilibrium. These include:

- Perception of the event by the individual
- The situational reports which are available
- Mechanisms of adaptation

The presence or absence of such factors will make all the difference in one's return to a state of equilibrium. The strength or weakness of one or more of these factors may be directly related to the initiation or resolution of a crisis.

A mechanical system is at equilibrium if the forces acting on it are in balance. For example, when a body floats, the force of gravity is balanced by the buoyant force due to displacement of the liquid. The "balance of nature" (Pimm, 1991) is an extension of this idea to the natural world. The concept usually refers to steady flows of energy and materials, rather than to a system whose components do not change.

Symptoms of Psychological Trauma

In a person's life when there occur events which threaten his/her biological, physical, or social wellbeing, there is a resulting disequilibrium. When this wellbeing is threatened, people react with anxiety. When there are a particularly large number of painful or unpleasant stimuli, like those associated with a disaster or tragedy, the individual requires a great capacity for adaptation. The mental health literature describes the stress following disaster and tragedy as a precise set of symptoms manifesting after an extraordinary traumatic event.

Symptoms of disaster-caused-stress will vary greatly, based on an individual's prior history of personal trauma, age, and ethnic background. Some of the typical symptoms experienced by both victims and responders are briefly described below.

- Individuals may have an exaggerated startle response or may exhibit hyper-vigilance. This is frequently seen after earthquakes, where people are known to jump in response to loud or sudden noises, such as doors slamming or trucks rumbling by.

- They may experience phobias about weather conditions (e.g., responses to wind noises following a tornado or hurricane) or other reminders that the accident or situation could happen again.

- They may experience difficulty with memory or calculations.

- Suddenly, they cannot balance their checkbook, or remember simple tasks, appointments, or such things as their address or phone number when asked.

- They may exhibit anger or even rage over their lack of control over the occurrence and their impotence at preventing it and protecting their families.

- Many times, this may be directed towards those who are trying to help.

BASIC-ID

Typical stress reactions to disaster trauma can be assessed by adopting the multi-modal behavioral approach initially outlined by Lazarus (1976, 1989, 2000). He used the acronym *BASIC-ID* to identify areas of concern for assessment. Responses generally assessed, using this model, are outlined below:

Behavioral Responses

- Hyper startle response
- Hyperactivity
- Workaholism
- Reckless, risk-taking behaviors
- Carelessness in tasks, leading to an increase in injuries
- Excessive use of sick leave
- Worried, rigid look, nervous activity
- Withdrawal or social isolation
- Inability to express self verbally or in writing
- Difficulty returning to normal activity
- Avoidance of places or activities that are reminders of the event
- Sexual problems

Affective/Emotional

- Initial euphoria and relief
- Survival guilt
- Anxiety, fear, insecurity
- Pervasive concern over the wellbeing of loved ones
- Feelings of helplessness, hopelessness
- Uncontrolled mood swings, periods of crying
- Apathy, isolation, detachment
- Shame or anger over vulnerability
- Irritability, restlessness, hyper-excitability, agitation
- Anger, rage, blame (often directed at those attempting to help)
- Frustration, cynicism, negativity
- Despair, grief, sadness
- Depression and withdrawal

Somatic/Sensation

- Vague body complaints
- Muscle aches and pains
- Fatigue or generalized weakness
- Sleep disturbances
- Increased or decreased heart rate or blood pressure
- Feeling of pounding heart or pulse
- Increase in allergies, colds, flu, headaches
- Trouble breathing or "getting breath"
- Tightness in chest, throat, or stomach
- Sweating
- Feeling of heaviness in arms or legs
- Numbness or tingling
- Changes in appetite or weight
- Nausea or GI (Gastrointestinal) upsets
- Trembling, dizziness or fainting

Imagery

- Sleep disturbances
- Nightmares
- Flashbacks and recurrent dreams of the event
- Intrusive thoughts about the event
- Ruminations about the event

Cognitive

- Inability to concentrate
- Difficulty with calculations
- Confusion, slowness of thought
- Impaired decision making
- Amnesia
- Preoccupation with the event
- Loss of objectivity
- Rigidity
- Loss of faith
- Increased awareness of one's own and loved ones' vulnerability
- Repetitive thoughts, memories, ruminations about the event
- Loss of judgment

Interpersonal Skills

- Irritability and anger toward others
- Family and relationship problems
- Disruption of work, school, or social relationships

Drugs/Alcohol

- Increased use of alcohol
- Increased use of drugs

Individuals exist in a normal state of "equilibrium" or balance. That emotional balance involves everyday stress, both positive and negative—like being late to work, getting a promotion, having a flat tire, getting ready for a date, or putting the children to bed. Occasionally, stress will be severe enough to move an individual out of his or her 'normal' state of equilibrium, and into a state of depression or anxiety. But most people, most of the time, stay in a familiar range of equilibrium.

When individuals are displaced from this equilibrium as a result of abrupt and strong changes (shocks, trauma) in the overall environment, wellbeing and happiness are affected. If the shock is positive (e.g., marriage, birth of a child, promotion, windfall inheritance), the individual experiences an increase in wellbeing. If the shock is negative (e.g., death of a child, parent or spouse, falling seriously ill, demotion, or getting fired), wellbeing is adversely affected.

Behavior adjusts to restore the individual to equilibrium through a combination of physical, emotional, behavioral, and psychological adjustments. This process of adjustment to external shocks/traumas creates physical, emotional, and psychological stress. This behavior implies that there is an optimum or equilibrium level of risk that people are generally comfortable with. If true, efforts to decrease risk may be met by riskier behavior.

Consider the case of farm tractors and road design. When tractors were designed for greater stability, farmers used them on steeper slopes and the accident rate remained constant. When highways were designed to be safer, drivers increased their speed and took more risks, and the accident rate remained at previous levels (Slovic, 1984). Ample evidence also illustrates that when individuals are placed in dangerous situations where there is risk of injury or death, they experience a higher level of stress (Seligman, 2004; Spitzer et al, 1005) which implies that they have the urge and motivation to take action to return to their equilibrium level of stress which is consistent with their desired comfort zone.

The nature of an individual's disposition also affects the rate of return to the equilibrium set point. For example, research suggests that optimistic patients live longer than pessimistic patients (Palmore, 1969a, 1969b). Happy people recover faster and some diseases can be cured or treated more effectively when the patient has a happy and upbeat attitude (Diener and Seligman, 2004). As a corollary to this, a pleasant mood seems to lower blood pressure and a high level of stress reduces the ability of the immune system to fight off disease. Furthermore, depression and anxiety, two major forms of mental illness, lead to significant decline in wellbeing (Spitzer et al, 1995; Packer, Husted, Cohen and Tomlinson, 1997). On the other hand, there is evidence that happy people show low signs of mental illness (Diener and Seligman, 2002). In addition, duration of unemployment and wellbeing are negatively related, and absenteeism and turnover rates are lower when workers are happier (Clegg, 1983; Clark, 2001; Akerlof et al, 1988).

There is also ample evidence that helping agents who experience negative shocks or trauma that reduce wellbeing make persistent attempts to return to equilibrium and to increase their levels of wellbeing and happiness. Those who are unemployed look for work. Those who are sick go to the doctor. Those who are divorced begin to date and often remarry. Those who move to a new city or neighborhood make efforts to make new friends. When life circumstances such as stress, trauma, critical incidents, war, death of relatives/close friends, and other negative developments disrupt this equilibrium, wellbeing is compromised.

According to Pimm (1991) and others, long may be indicative of a loss of resilience. Pimm is concerned with behavior near a stable equilibrium. In that case, a long return time for a given displacement from the equilibrium indicates a small coefficient or, equivalently, a small derivative. Others are concerned with behavior of a system with two or three equilibria, one of which is stable. Resilience describes the tendency of the system to return to its stable equilibrium. A long return time is due to disturbances that bring the system near an unstable equilibrium, or possibly, to a weak repulsion from an unstable equilibrium. Analysis suggests that happiness over time varies directly and significantly with several dimensions of people's lives including family life, health, work, and social environment (Easterlin, 2004).

Life disruptions have a strong negative and very strong impact on happiness and wellbeing. Social mobility as reflected by the number of moves also has a significant impact on wellbeing. Making more moves tends to reduce trust, while fewer moves tend to increase trust and cohesion in neighborhoods. Twenge (2002) and Magdol (2002) conclude that frequent moves have a detrimental impact on families, particularly in wives. Long-distance mobility discourages individuals in forming long-lasting community ties and has a negative impact on wellbeing. Illness, mental anguish, and death in families also have a very strong negative impact on wellbeing (Di Tella et al, 2003; Layard, 2005; Diener and Seligman, 2004). Disruption in the form of vulnerabilities to floods, hurricanes, earthquakes, tornadoes, and other natural disasters also results in lower levels of wellbeing (Veenhoven, 1994).

Poor health and illness diminishes wellbeing quite dramatically as shown in several studies (World Values Study Group, 1994; Packer, Husted, Cohen and Tomlinson, 1997; Diener and Seligman, 2004; Gerlach and Stephan, 1996). Depression and other psychiatric illness together make up about 30 percent of the various causes of disability. This is a much higher rate than disability from alcohol and drug addiction making 10%, respiratory illness, cancer and heart trouble making 15% (Layard, 2005, Chapter 11). There is also evidence that happy people show fewer signs of mental illness (Diener and Seligman, 2004).

Rewarding social interactions are key components of wellbeing (Baumeister and Leary, 1995). This entails frequent and pleasant interactions with a few people within the context of a stable, trusting, and mutual relationship and providing a stronger and more substantive bond and feeling of belonging than one based on self-interest alone (Clark, 1984; Clark and Mills, 1979). Superficial social contacts cannot substitute for deeper and more intimate relationships (Weiss, 1973); Baumeister and Leary, 1995). Positive social bonds are associated with positive emotions and higher levels of wellbeing (See Sternberg, 1986 and McAdams, 1985). Conversely, the loss of friends leads to loneliness and depression (Leary, 1990) as well as anxiety (Baumeister and Tice, 1990). Other research shows that intimate relationships and close social and family ties are highly valued by respondents and, in the case of sexual intimacy, result in a significantly high increase in wellbeing (Kahneman, Krueger, Schkade, Schwartz, and Stone, 2004; Diener and Seligman, 2002; Blanchflower and Oswald, 2003). The death of a spouse, child, or close friend ranks high on the list of stressful and difficult events and can result in a period of depression (Holmes and Rahe, 1967; Weiss, 1979).

When trauma occurs, people are thrown so far out of the range of equilibrium that it is difficult for them to restore a sense of balance in life. Trauma may be precipitated by stress "acute" or "chronic". Acute stress is usually caused by a sudden, arbitrary, often random event. Chronic stress is one that occurs over and over again—each time pushing the individual toward the edge of his or her state of equilibrium or beyond. Most trauma comes from acute, unexpected stressors, such as violent crime, natural disasters, accidents, or acts of war. Some trauma is caused by quite predictable (but hated) stressors, such as the chronic abuse of a child, spouse, or elder.

Before a disaster occurs, the majority of people are usually in a state of relative equilibrium. When a stressful incident occurs, people experience a state of disequilibrium and there is a perceived need to return to equilibrium. Faced with this dynamic situation, the role of mental health professionals and related responders is to support and, at the same time, accelerate the re-equilibrium process. Thus, the worker may have to deal with disaster victims who are in various states of recovery. On the one hand, there are those who, because of the presence of compensation factors, situational support, and appropriate adaptation mechanisms, have a realistic perception of the incident. This usually leads to resolution as one's equilibrium is regained without crisis. On the other hand, there are others who, because of the absence of compensation factors, of situational support, and of adaptive mechanisms, may have a distorted perception of the incident. Problems then remain unresolved, resulting in disequilibrium and crisis. A crisis intervention referral is needed (Aguilera and Messick, 1976).

When a disaster or other critical incident occurs, people are traumatized at different levels, mostly dependent upon how directly affected they are. Much effort and much discussion often revolves around returning to normal. However, "normal" has changed. It is a concept with many different meanings. It tends to be a term that is very difficult to define and, consequently, implement. What was "normal" before can never be the same again. What can happen and what is constructive, and more easily defined, is a "Return to Equilibrium". This involves integrating the event, its effects and its meaning, into one's life, and recognizing it as now part of one's life. Taking that and building a new balance in life can bring one into a new and enriched life. To use a concrete example, it is quite akin to taking an old fashioned balance and adding or subtracting to one side or another in order to gain a balanced scale. Experience in life changes each of us whether the experience is good or bad. Integrating that experience into our life creates that new balance. It is a changed normality that results from the new balance and a return to equilibrium.

Returning to equilibrium following a major hurricane or other natural event is different from returning to equilibrium following a man-made traumatic event, critical incident, terrorism event, or war. However, in all cases, re-establishing a balance in life that integrates the event as part of one's life and moving forward into the future in a constructive manner is what develops our new "normality". Such a "Return to Equilibrium" is a goal of recovery.

A stress response that fails to return to a state of equilibrium becomes unresolved psychological/emotional trauma. Emotional or psychological trauma is the extreme end of the stress disorder continuum. It is stress run amuck—a deregulation of the nervous system that remains fixed and contributes to lifelong mental, emotional, and physical disorders including anxiety and depression. Emotional or psychological trauma can result from such common occurrences as an auto accident, the breakup of a significant relationship, a humiliating or deeply disappointing experience, the discovery of a life-threatening illness or disabling condition, or other similar situations. Traumatizing events can take a serious emotional toll on those involved, even if the event did not cause physical damage.

Conclusions

Following a disaster, it is common for individuals to feel pressure to reduce distressing emotions brought on by the event and return to adaptive, independent, everyday functioning. For first responders, returning to everyday functioning involves managing residual effects from the disaster, being able to handle the day-to-day stressors of work, and being prepared to respond to any future crisis. First responders may want to avoid talking about the disaster. Avoidance can also take on other forms, such as missing work or even working too much. Although avoidant strategies may be initially highly adaptive, allowing the first responder to continue working, continuous use or overuse of avoidance can impede long-term positive readjustment. An active problem-solving approach that actively addresses difficulties posed by the stressor can help with both chronic and acute stressors. For example, finding meaning in some outcome of the disaster may minimize feelings of helplessness, instill a sense of control and mastery, and is typically associated with better physical and psychological outcomes than avoidant coping.

Following an intensely stressful event, first responders may believe that by talking about the event, they will burden family and friends, or that other people "just don't understand." However, talking about, or even writing about, the experience can be healthy and therapeutic. Discussing the event does not need to take place immediately following the stressful experience. Judgment should guide the decision to whom and when to open up. If a trusted confidante extends an offer to listen and discuss the experience and reactions to the disaster, and the first responder desires to talk about his or her experiences, this might be beneficial. If, on the other hand, first responders are not yet ready to discuss their experiences, their decision should be respected. It is important that all relationships be built upon communications, also allowing the right to not communicate. It is helpful, however, for first responders to remember to keep their options open and to let those who have offered their support at least know that their offer has been heard and appreciated. This is especially true with family members.

Every time a stressful event happens, there are certain recognized compensating factors which can help promote a return to equilibrium. These include:

- Perception of the event by the individual
- The situational reports which are available
- Mechanisms of adaptation

The presence or absence of such factors will make all the difference in one's return to a state of equilibrium, The strength or weakness of one or more of these factors may be directly related to the initiation or resolution of a crisis.

When stress originates externally, internal changes occur. This is why certain events can cause a strong emotional reaction in one person and leave another indifferent. Crisis Counseling Programs can play a very important role in helping rural families to assess the issues involved and make good decisions regarding their immediate and long-term needs.

5 Meeting the Challenges

The economic farm crisis of the late 1970s and early 1980s graphically demonstrated the interconnection between the farm community and the small towns and cities that comprise rural areas. When the farm community suffers, agriculture-related businesses suffer as well. The impact continues to grocery stores, clothing stores, restaurants, churches, and it flows through the entire community. The following excerpt from *Taking Rural Into Account: Report on the National Public Forum* (CMHS, 1993) provides an excellent summary regarding challenges of healthcare in general and mental healthcare in particular in the rural areas of our nation:

> Rural Americans experience incidence and prevalence rates of mental illness, substance abuse, emotional disturbance, and developmental disability equal to or greater than their urban counterparts. Yet only 25 percent of the rural poor qualify for Medicaid compared to 43 percent of the poor in inner cities (Special Committee on Aging, United States Senate, 1988).

The rural population has a disproportionate number of poor elderly, children and adolescents, minorities, and migrant workers, who are at high risk for mental disorders. Despite this reality, the public mental health system is often the only mental health provider in rural areas. Sixty-one percent of rural Americans live in designated psychiatric-shortage areas (U.S. Congress, 1988). As a result, rural individuals often have to travel long distances to obtain services or depend on providers who travel periodically to rural areas. This means that rural individuals frequently do not get the help they need, or they wait until they are in a crisis situation.

Finally, the impact of a disaster in an area where agriculture accounts for a major portion of the local economy may not be evident until months after the event. The impact on planting and harvest seasons, erosion of the topsoil, contaminants, and fluctuations in market prices combine to form an economic crisis. The economic impact on agribusiness is impossible to measure in the first several weeks or months after the declaration. Farmers may not apply for assistance or underestimate their need if they do apply. Stress is generated by:

- Uncertainty (level of crop damage, price fluctuations, etc.)
- Time limits on applying for assistance
- The culture, competition, and beliefs on self-reliance as a measure of worth
- Distrust of outsiders and government intervention
- A maze of programs, red tape, and paperwork in the disaster recovery process

The Crisis Counseling Program can play a very important role in helping rural families to assess the issues involved and make good decisions regarding their immediate and long-term needs.

Challenges Encountered by Rural Crisis Counseling Programs

Crisis counseling staff responding to a rural disaster faces unique challenges related to the values and characteristics of rural areas and people discussed in Chapter Two. Planning and persistence may help to overcome some of the challenges associated with rural areas. Recommendations are provided on how to reach farm families, people who are emotionally isolated and independent, and how to overcome constraints of geographic isolation and access hard to reach groups.

Emotional Isolation and Independence of the Rural Population

Initial contact may reveal a person or family caught in an angry reaction to a multitude of aggravations. Doors may be slammed and workers may bear the brunt of yelling and abusive language. While forcing the issue is never appropriate, a contact later in the program may reveal a completely different temperament. A person who was completely closed at a prior point may, in a few short days or weeks, be open to contact and appreciative of services. Phases of recovery shift and change. As trust begins to develop, people gradually become receptive to the efforts of outreach workers. Over the long haul, outreach workers gain respect for their willingness and tenacity from the people they have attempted to serve.

Reaching Farm Families

The Crisis Counseling Programs that were successful with rural outreach to farm families were those that had the assistance of organizations experienced in dealing with farm families and farm issues. One such group, the Farm Resource Center in Illinois, has been operational since the early 1980s providing families with crisis counseling, financial planning assistance, and referrals to other programs. The experience of the Farm Resource Center's workers served as a model to crisis counselors on how outreach is conducted in the farm community.

Other Midwest States used similar organizations with connections to the farm community to open the door to outreach efforts. Many contacts and services were facilitated by these working relationships. This is further reinforcement of the principle that no matter what type of group a program is attempting to reach, finding outreach workers representative of that group is the best way to gain access.

Geographic Isolation

Geography's role in rural crisis counseling is significant. It often takes days to accomplish the same number of outreach contacts one can make in an afternoon in an urban area. Traveling from place to place can be difficult, given the disaster's impact on roads and bridges. A rural outreach worker needs information from State and county highway departments and law enforcement officials to stay current on conditions. Detailed topographical maps may be available from the FEMA Disaster Field Office or State Emergency Management Office.

An outreach worker's inability to reach some impacted people often means that the survivors themselves cannot get out except with four-wheel drive vehicles. Such isolation creates difficulty getting into town, getting children to school, and perhaps most important, obtaining food and medical care. In many rural areas, emergency medical services are not immediately available.

Basic access issues can be a consideration, such as getting to the grocery store, gasoline station, bank, and other businesses following a disaster. During the height of the '93 Midwest floods, thirty-minute commutes to work and school became two hours and longer due to washed out roads and bridges (Project Recovery Final Report, Illinois, 1994). Because of the distances involved and lack of easy access, rural residents may forgo attending meetings or accessing services at some "in-town" location. Consequently, support groups, educational events, and other group services may not be the best option in some areas. Most counseling will take place at the disaster survivor's home rather than at an office.

Many addresses are only listed by a rural route number or a post office box number. Locating the home of such a person means developing a good set of directions. Information from local officials about access problems, as well as information about the physical characteristics of the location, such as color of the house, type of siding, and model of parked automobiles, may be the only way to find the correct dwelling. In addition, the presence of outbuildings and large landmarks, such as grain silos or dairy storage tanks, can be a valuable identifier in locating the right farm or homestead.

Many people served by rural programs are at or below the poverty level. Finding people who do not have a telephone is common. Contact with such people to see if they are home before making the trip may be difficult if there is not a neighbor or family member close by to relay information. While mail contact is possible, it takes more time and is not responsive to short-term emergency needs. Also, literacy levels should be considered in the development of any mailing, flyers, and outreach educational materials.

Accessing Hard-to-Reach Groups

Some organizations, such as those working on healthcare, child welfare, and schools, function in a somewhat self-contained environment. Though such an organizational structure does not render interagency communication impossible, it does make access a challenge. The following strategies may assist rural crisis counseling projects in providing a wide array of services to these hard-to-access groups:

Do Your Homework

Before making the first contact, find out as much as possible about the organization and the best person to contact. With this information, developing a presentation or package of services that will be received positively may be feasible.

Develop a Personal Contact

Trust and confidence, especially in programs that are new and time-limited, such as disaster crisis counseling, must be built person-to-person. People in rural areas refer to other people more often than to programs. The person who is a primary contact may not be the person who has authority to invite crisis counseling services into the organization. Having someone who can exert influence from within can result in the decision maker contacting the outreach worker to request services.

Knowing people's names also provides a point of contact in case there are difficulties or miscommunications. Being able to pick up the phone and call a person you know by name, have met face to face, and have established a working relationship with is a tremendous asset to an outreach worker.

Hire Outreach Workers or Volunteers who Have Worked in the Organization or Field that is Difficult to Penetrate

Certain groups or organizations will be key to the success of the outreach effort. In the rural area, schools and agricultural and religious groups and organizations are especially helpful. Hiring staff that knows those groups, and better yet are known by them, can help get quick and effective outreach efforts into those groups.

Hiring a retired school administrator, teacher, or counselor to do outreach can provide a natural relationship to access schools. Some agricultural groups may be difficult to access unless the crisis counseling project has farmers or university extension personnel either doing outreach or assisting outreach workers in meeting farm families in need. In Ventura County, California, the Northridge earthquake survivors included non-English speaking families and migrant workers with minimal education. Language, low-literacy, isolation, and the fear and anxiety of deportation presented challenging barriers for the outreach workers to overcome. The crisis counseling project assigned bilingual, bicultural staff, and provided door-to-door outreach to identify the specific needs of the survivor. Linking disaster survivors to counseling services with trusted church and community-based organizations was also a successful service delivery method. The church is an effective catalyst in the provision of services to these special populations. Churches have historically been a place where migrant workers and monolingual families feel comfortable in seeking services (Northridge Earthquake Final Report, Ventura County, California, 1995).

Use Easy-to-Reach Groups to Reach Hard-to-Reach Groups

Sometimes crisis counselors will not make the first contact. An organization already working cooperatively with the crisis counseling project can provide great assistance in influencing other groups. By conveying a sense of the nature, importance, and credibility of the crisis counseling effort, these partners can help unlock new opportunities for outreach.

Do What You Can, When You Can

If a full range of outreach services are not what an organization or group desires, provide what they are willing to accept. Perhaps all that can be done is distribute materials or give an educational presentation. Just as people progress through phases of recovery, so do organizations. Maintaining contact at any level may result in more significant services later as the organization's needs become more apparent or change with time.

Crisis Counseling Programs for the Rural Community

Coordinating Services: Working with Existing Resources

The organizational structures of rural crisis counseling projects are as varied as the States and communities affected. Flexibility and creativity are highly valued components of a rural crisis counseling project. In a rural area, where there are fewer organized and structured resources, the program must adapt, invent, and convert itself fully to utilize existing resources and to fulfill the mission of the program. How the goals are accomplished and how those outcomes are achieved differ for each program.

Networking gives crisis counseling workers ready access to staff of other programs. Referrals can be made and a good working relationship can develop as a result. Endorsement of the outreach effort also increases the level of investment that leaders have in the project. That investment will often carry over to a higher regard for other mental health programs. The following are examples of how rural programs can work with existing resources.

Crisis Counseling Training for Gatekeepers

Mental health needs in a rural community are addressed by more than just local mental health professionals. Clergy, school counselors, physicians, healthcare workers, welfare workers, funeral directors, and many other gatekeepers are a vital part of the rural community's support system. Some of these individuals, by virtue of their role in the community, may have awareness of people who have not yet come into contact with the crisis counseling project. Apprising these people of crisis counseling services and offering training on disaster mental health, basic crisis intervention, and counseling skills is prudent. Because the gatekeepers may come into contact with disaster survivors who need more intensive mental health services, the training needs to include procedures for referrals.

Consultation

Some people may be actively involved in providing support and care to others who simply need to discuss the disaster's impact with someone trained in disaster mental health. Outreach workers can provide valuable consultation to these people in helping them understand the normal, expected responses to the disaster. Agencies and institutions may also need consultation to help them assist their staff and clients. Existing social and human service agencies, as well as groups that were formed as part of the disaster recovery effort, are examples of agencies that may benefit from consultation. Outreach efforts for formal agencies are similar to those provided to the natural network of gatekeepers. Provide information on what is normal and predictable, as well as when and where to seek help and from whom.

Community Organization

The important role the community plays in the daily life of the rural disaster survivor makes it essential for outreach workers to participate in committees and other community structures as part of the disaster response and recovery effort. This participation gives continuous opportunity for the workers to keep other key people and programs updated on the crisis counseling services. Also, serving on committees provides opportunity for the workers to know the status of other relief efforts, how to access the various resources, and where there may be pockets of unreached individuals. The restoration of natural networks and support systems must be addressed on a community-wide basis. Information and handouts on disaster recovery phases and disaster mental health response issues can greatly enhance planning efforts.

Referral Options

Some individuals will experience significant emotional distress, even at the time the program is closing. These people may need a referral for traditional mental healthcare. This can be a sensitive issue in rural communities and should be addressed in crisis counseling training during the preparation for program closure. The rural attitudes and unique characteristics of the service area will affect how people respond to a mental health referral. Often, options for making an effective mental health referral may be limited. In particular, inpatient care may be difficult to access. Specialized care for children, substance abuse problems, and many other issues requiring unique treatment programs may be located more than 100 miles away.

Being well-acquainted with the intake and/or treatment staff of the local community mental health provider(s) is important for the crisis counseling staff. In addition, the mental health provider should know and have a working relationship with other programs whose services may be helpful to disaster survivors.

Networking with Community Resources

To be effective, rural crisis counseling projects must establish themselves in the mix of programs and organizations active in the disaster response (See Appendix for a listing of organizations and resources involved in disaster response and recovery). Identifying what other resources and services are available is essential to providing good information to recipients of outreach. Providing information to other programs and services about the crisis counseling project extends the efforts of outreach staff and results in referrals. Interagency meetings provide information on the current status of services, changes in programs, and referral criteria. These meetings may also provide an opportunity to problem-solve where difficulties may have developed in working relationships.

Sharing a Meal

It is important to understand that in rural areas, a shared meal can be a powerful conduit to interaction and problem-solving among disaster survivors, community leaders, and crisis counselors. Although Federal regulations and FEMA policy do not allow crisis counseling funds to be spent on entertainment, rural crisis counseling projects have successfully brought survivors and community resources together for meetings with food served using the following strategies:

- Encourage potluck meals held at a neutral community site such as a community center, school, or church. Such meals can precede/follow support group meetings or community forums featuring such speakers as FEMA, unmet needs committee representatives, local, State, or Federal government representatives, or outreach workers. Such potluck events can be creatively organized around themes, such as desserts only, with donations to cover coffee.

- Organize donated meals provided by community groups or local service organizations for the same purposes as listed above. Such organizations may actually cook meals (chili supper, pancake breakfast) on-site for the meeting participants. One Midwestern community held monthly support group meetings at local restaurants. The restaurant meeting site changed monthly. Each month a different service group paid for the meals. It was also a boon for the local business owners who hosted these groups at their dining establishment.

- Dutch treat meals can be successful if the price is reasonable. Groups can either meet at a local restaurant or have a local caterer provide the food. Keeping costs low is best. Do not rule out breakfast meetings if that is a good time for survivors to participate. Remember that lunch is usually less expensive than an evening meal.

Offering coffee and cookies or some type of shared meal can facilitate disaster survivor interaction and participation in community forums, support groups, etc., in rural communities. Local programs can be as creative as possible to provide food for these meetings while adhering to FEMA crisis counseling regulations.

Religious Groups and Clergy

The ability to provide information regarding disaster crisis counseling services to a wide cross-section of the community is enhanced greatly by working with and through the various churches and religious organizations in a community. Working as an ally with church groups can open the way for outreach to many families. Religious groups can mobilize many people and are fertile soil for finding volunteers. The benevolent work of such groups can provide an effective alternative to the outreach worker becoming over involved in the issues of shelter, clothing, and financial resources. Religious organizations, such as interfaith groups and ministerial alliances, can ensure a coordinated and comprehensive effort within the religious community.

One by-product of involvement with church groups is the ability to reach several age groups in one setting. There also may be church groups for specific ages. In addition, each person in the groups has his or her own network of family, friends, and co-workers who might also benefit from crisis counseling services.

In areas where cultural and ethnic populations reside, the church may be the one source of contact trusted by the community as a whole. The lack of trust or confidence a person has for local, State, or Federal government can create a barrier to receiving much needed assistance. The barrier can often be overcome by involving a church or other community organization that the disaster survivor trusts.

Pastors, rabbis, and clergy may need crisis counseling themselves. Religious leaders are often stretched to the limit with their congregation's post-disaster needs. An added stressor may be the financial health of the parish due to reduced income of members. Provide clergy members information on key concepts of disaster mental health, stress management, and anniversary reactions. This information can be used for sermons, as inserts in the church program or bulletin and posted on parish bulletin boards.

Community Groups

Crisis counseling projects should work with community groups by providing information on common disaster mental health reactions, the services available through the crisis counseling project, and how to obtain additional information. The following list of community groups in a rural area can assist in identifying people needing crisis counseling:

- Local American Red Cross
- Salvation Army
- City or Regional Development Corporations
- Agricultural Soil Conservation Service (ASCS)
- Veterinarians
- City and County Government
- Mail carriers
- Funeral directors
- Cooperative Extension Offices
- Farm Organizations such as National Farmers Organization (NFO), Farm Bureau, Farmer's Aid and Farm Resource Center
- Churches
- Ministerial Alliance
- Native American Groups
- Migrant Worker Services

- Local Immigrant Groups and Organizations
- Clubs such as: Lions, Rotary, Kiwanis, Civitan, Ruritan, Elks, Eagles, and Oddfellows
- Business and Professional Women (BPW)
- Women's Sororities
- Chambers of Commerce
- Child Welfare Agencies
- Pre-schools, Day Care Centers, Head Start Programs, and Birth to Three Programs
- Schools, Public and Private including Junior Colleges, Colleges and Universities
- Hospitals
- Senior and low income housing
- Rural Health Clinics
- Substance Abuse Treatment Facilities
- Alcohol and Drug Prevention Education Programs
- Physicians, Dentists, Chiropractors
- Home Health Agencies
- Visiting Nurse Association (VNA)
- Pharmacists
- Seniors programs
- Seed corn dealers
- Farm implement dealers
- Battery and tire businesses
- Insurance offices
- Banks and other lending businesses
- Employment Security Office
- Public Assistance Office
- Public Health Department

- Vocational Rehabilitation
- Developmental Disabilities Services
- Nursing homes and sheltered care facilities
- Barbers and beauticians
- Restaurants and coffee shops
- Home delivery sales people
- Utility meter readers
- Catholic Social Services
- Lutheran Social Services

The list could go on and on. In each rural community, there are unique groups and organizations that can assist in identifying disaster survivors in need of crisis counseling services.

Special Community Services

Community Healing Events

In a rural community, the recovery of individual disaster survivors is greatly impacted by the community's ability to heal. Around the one-year anniversary of the disaster, residents may plan a variety of community events to commemorate the disaster. Often such events commemorate the casualties of disaster, celebrate the recovery, and show appreciation for those who helped others. A single event may be able to reach a whole rural community or several smaller events may be organized. When the timing is right and there is broad community interest, involvement, and support, community events can be a powerful force in bringing closure coupled with positive anticipation for the future. Commonly, these events will express "how far we have come" since the disaster's onset. The event is an opportunity to bring together the rural community that may have been dispersed due to housing shortages and changes in employment.

Crisis counseling workers must remember that while most of the community may be ready and interested in a "healing event", not everyone will share this desire. Some people may not feel like celebrating or coming together. These people may experience a heightened sense of isolation from their neighbors and friends due to this difference. They may fear that something is wrong with them since everyone else seems ready to get on with their lives. Sensitivity to these different feelings is an important way the crisis counseling project can ensure that it is responsive to everyone, no matter where they are in the recovery process (CMHS, 1994).

Prior to the anniversary date, there may be symbolic and ceremonial expressions of grief and support. These may be organized, but more often occur spontaneously. They may be more isolated expressions of individuals or small groups and not the wider community. There is a healing impact in such expressions that may pave the way for the healing of the community as a whole. Being sensitive to the use of terminology is also important. A "commemoration" may be considered more appropriate than a "celebration".

Crisis counselors can provide helpful consultation to community groups considering such events, and can be useful in helping to coordinate and implement them. Running the show is seldom useful for the crisis counseling project unless requested by the community.

Continued Access to Needed Services

At program close, it is important that clear communication take place with other community programs working cooperatively with the crisis counseling effort. These community programs can be of valuable assistance in identifying other support services and individuals that can serve as resources. Many people in rural communities do not know what services are available or from whom. Crisis counseling staff can inform local programs of what type and degree of continued mental health support will be available to the community through the local mental health provider. All recipients of the crisis counseling services need to be notified that they will be referred to local/regional resources if there is continuing need.

Flyers or brochures outlining existing resources for various types of human service needs should be prepared. Public education can be provided to civic groups and businesses. Public service announcements about the closing of the project can get the word out and be used for expressions of thanks to the various people and organizations in the community who have supported the program. Disseminating information regarding human service assistance programs is always important.

Recognition and Appreciation

During the closing weeks, program coordinators and administrators should express appreciation and provide recognition to those people in the community who assisted the crisis counseling project. Letters of thanks, not only to the people themselves but to the supervisor or the director of their organization, can communicate such appreciation. Recognition at a public meeting with appreciation letters or certificates can be effective.

A by-product of this effort is continued good working relationships beyond the disaster. Most of the organizations and people who have provided crisis counseling services during the months of the program will continue to work and live in the same communities. The cooperative spirit and mutual appreciation that existed during the disaster recovery effort carries over in many cases to the ongoing working relationships.

There are many examples of interagency groups that began to meet because of disaster and continued well after other recovery efforts were done. They continued in this fashion, not out of reluctance to let go of the disaster, but because they found the networking and information sharing at such meetings to be essential to their more routine working relationships.

Rural Crisis Counseling Project Staff

Recruitment and Staffing

The quality of staff and their understanding of the program are essential to the success of the rural crisis counseling project. Staffing issues that impact rural crisis counseling projects include the pool of individuals available for hire, the hiring of people representative of the population to be served, and their responsiveness to training and supervision. The following generalizations regarding staffing can be made based on the experience of past rural disaster projects:

Previous Disaster Experience

If workers are hired from the impacted area, the majority will not have had experience working in a disaster relief program. Some may have personal disaster-related life experience, but working with this program will be their first formal involvement. This lack of experience places a great deal of importance on the areas of training, supervision, and staff support.

Outreach Staff Characteristics

Rural disaster programs use a high percentage of local people in their outreach and crisis counseling efforts. Almost without exception, the use of indigenous workers is integral to program success. Project COPE in Ventura County, California, enlisted people with serious and persistent mental illness to perform outreach to other people affected by the disaster who had a mental illness. This approach was highly successful (Northridge Earthquake Final Report, Ventura County, California, 1995).

Rural outreach workers often have a car as their office, find themselves making contacts with people they already know, and often receive calls at home at all hours. Consistent training and supervision on managing these unusual circumstances are necessary not only to protect the wellbeing of the worker, but to protect the worker's family functioning as well.

Small Towns and Country Areas

In many rural agencies and organizations, it is more likely that one will know or have some acquaintance with the people contacted. This familiarity provides a greater sense of safety and assurance for the worker in making the rounds from house to house or farm to farm. It may also present concerns about dual relationships, boundaries, and limits.

Volunteers

People who wish to be of assistance to the outreach effort on a non-paid basis still need training and supervision. It is important that they understand the nature, scope, and limitations of the program and the means by which services can be delivered. There are dozens of ways outreach staff can use the assistance of volunteers in conducting community education, outreach to children, distributing materials, and other activities.

Screening Volunteer and Paid Staff

A careful screening, interview, and reference check process before accepting an individual as part of the program are critical. In rural communities, word travels extremely fast. If the crisis counseling project has an outreach worker or volunteer who is inappropriate or a poor representative of the program, the community's confidence in the program will plummet quickly.

Training and Ongoing Supervision

No matter who is hired, what their background or experience, they will need training and supervision to be a productive member of the crisis counseling project. Licensed clinicians and professionals require orientation to crisis counseling concepts, and therefore must be expected to receive the same training as paraprofessionals or non-licensed individuals (NIMH, 1983).

In addition, staff may benefit from specialized training that reflects the nature of the work in rural areas. Safety and security issues and cultural sensitivity training may be as important as basic disaster stress training. Some issues to consider are:

Cultural Sensitivity Regarding New or Transient Residents in the Area

Small towns are sometimes attractive to groups of immigrants such as Laotian, Cambodian, Somalian, or Vietnamese. Migrant populations also pose cultural barriers or social nuances that can impact a worker's acceptance as a helper.

Special population groups may also inhabit rural areas. Crisis counseling workers should be briefed on any group of people who may pose a challenge or threat to them. Rural areas are popular with extremist groups, and are potential sites for production of illegal crops.

Crisis communication and conflict resolution skills are important in a rural setting because workers are often alone and may be in remote areas. Consideration should be given to providing training on self-defense strategies. Many police departments will provide training in defensive tactics for little or no fee. Every worker should know the emergency resources available (sheriff, emergency medical services, and crisis intervention services) in their region and have immediate access via cellular phones or two way radios.

Tips and techniques for managing a confrontation with an angry dog may help prepare workers to deal with a threatening situation. Further, consider the types of wildlife that may be encountered in a crisis counseling staff's travels. Training on identifying and managing situations in which workers may encounter dangerous wildlife—such as poisonous snakes, alligators, moose, bears, or tics that produce Lyme Disease—may help prevent injury.

"How to talk to farmers" may be helpful training for workers unfamiliar with the jargon regarding agricultural areas. A primer on hog farming, sugar beets, or peach orchards may help workers connect by speaking the same language. The university extension or agricultural service agencies in most States may be able to help with this type of training.

Staff Safety and Security

Staff safety and security is always a concern for crisis counseling projects. Concerns that have impacted rural crisis counseling projects are centered on three main areas:

- Workers becoming stranded

- Natural risks such as dogs, physical exhaustion, and illness
- The risk of personal harm from individuals due to anger, substance abuse, or other factors that increase the potential for violence

Workers Becoming Stranded

Outreach workers for past programs have worked alone and in pairs. Male/female teams have proven successful. Workers have reported a greater sense of security and less isolation by working in pairs. Also, disaster survivors were not as wary of a couple as they might be of two men. Female outreach workers felt safer working in tandem with a male co-worker. Dual-gender teams allowed natural access to the husband/farmer and the wife/homemaker.

Traveling late in the day to early evening was a concern for some outreach workers, particularly in winter when the weather is unpredictable. Providing cellular phones helped with communication. Establishing specific times for workers to call into the office each day not only addressed safety concerns, but also improved communication with the office and survivors (Project Help Final Report, Wisconsin, 1994). In areas where a worker may be far from home at the end of a day of outreach, budgeting for some overnight lodging can decrease night driving, save time, and decrease wear-and-tear on the worker, as well as address safety issues. The cell phone programs provided a way to maintain contact with workers. A routine opportunity to debrief by sharing concerns and feelings associated with the day-to-day aspects of the job also provided supervisory and administrative staff feedback on what might be done to improve the safety of the workers. It is also an important opportunity for the worker to connect with other staff and process their feelings.

Natural Risks

When an outreach worker gets out of the automobile at a farm house, there could very well be several dogs, not just one. Training on how to respond to agitated animals by a professional animal handler would be an unusual, but useful, addition to a program where these risks exist.

Other natural risks relate to the potential for injury, stress-related ailments, and other health difficulties in outreach staff. Working long hours, exposure to the elements, and contact with large numbers of disaster survivors, can lower resistance to illness such as influenza. Crisis counseling staff tends to be very good at taking care of others but not as good at taking care of themselves. Rotating workers out of a disaster soon after the immediate impact is a way of avoiding burnout in disaster responders. Even over the longer term of the Regular Services project, rotating workers out of the disaster-affected area periodically can help reduce stress levels and provide a refreshing change of pace. In a rural setting, the isolation and overwork, rather than the overwhelming scenes of disaster impact, create problems.

Staff needs to know that such periodic breaks from the intensity of their daily work are essential and required by supervisors. Such involvement both enhances their personal health and their ability to do good work. Injury is a risk due to the state of disrepair of many areas where rural outreach takes place. Debris and broken items in and around a home and ongoing construction projects constitute the greatest risks. Outreach workers should have a current tetanus shot (within ten years). The presence of foreign objects in roadways increases the potential for flat tires and automobile accidents. Training on how to reduce risks of personal injury can create a climate of safety consciousness and, hopefully, reduce adverse incidents to workers during the program.

Risk of Harm from Others

By the very nature of the program, there is risk that an outreach worker will meet one or more individuals who are frustrated, angry, and stressed. Some rural residents have purposely isolated themselves from others and may not be receptive to a home visit. Some people, even before the disaster, are antisocial and intimidating. Still others may be self-medicating for stress with alcohol or other drugs, escalating their potential for violence. The potential of encountering these individuals is a concern for outreach worker safety.

Workers need to understand that they may seek the assistance of law enforcement any time they feel their physical safety is at risk. Since contact with such aid may not be readily available in the midst of the situation, workers need to know it is all right to leave at any point if their concern begins to rise. Personal safety training may be beneficial. Providing guidance on signs of agitation and emotional difficulty, along with non-physical techniques for a de-escalation of such circumstances, is very useful. As noted earlier, consider providing cellular phones or even two-way radios to outreach workers.

Outreach staff should have a clear protocol of how to respond when in a physically threatening situation. They should carry the names and numbers of law enforcement and mental health crisis intervention programs that may be used in an emergency. Consult with local law enforcement authorities and crisis intervention programs.

Rural Mental Health Centers

Rural Clinics Mental Health Centers continue to provide a comprehensive array of services to the Severely Mentally Ill (SMI) adult and Severely Emotionally Disturbed (SED) children populations.

Outpatient counseling (individual, family, and group), Psychosocial Rehabilitation, Case Management, Medication Clinics, Residential Supports, and Mental Health Court are often available at Satellite and Sub-Satellite Clinics. Emergency services are provided, including co-occurring substance abuse programs in some areas. Services are generally available for all persons who qualify regardless of their ability to pay. Insurance, Medicare, Medicaid fee, and sliding fee scale may be accepted. Rural Clinics and Mental Health Centers continue efforts towards application to and attainment of accreditations.

This website provides an example of statewide Rural Mental Health Clinics: http://mhds.nv.gov/index.php?option=com_content&task=view&id=31&Itemid=64

Some Cross-Cultural Differences

The environment is the source of many stressors which can initiate a variety of reactions. These reactions may range from endocrine secretions to such things as complicated appraisals and evaluations of the sources. These reactions to stressors may be physiological (Selye, 1956/1976) and/or psychological (Lazarus, 1966; Lazarus and Cohen, 1977; Lazarus and Launier, 1978). Few investigators have attempted to study all aspects of the stress process simultaneously.

Stressful responses can be evoked by the changes and challenges that one experiences in daily life. They can be caused by the disruption of one's habits (e.g., unpredictable noise or crowding). Malfunctioning of social systems which place obstacles in one's path, deprivation, losses, and culturally-governed mores may also contribute to stressful responses. Stressors may be intrusive, physical and universally threatening (e.g. natural disasters). Others may be more culturally determined, less universal, and more psychosocial in nature. Aiello and Thompson (1980) and Hall (1966) found that varying intensities of crowding and proximities in spatial invasion are specific to cultural norms and meanings.

The obvious lack of relative crowding and the presence of generous open space in western rural areas would seem to offer escape from the stressors generally associated with urban areas. The lessening of noise factors, crowding, and other variables associated with stress production would seem to enhance the quality of life. In fact, these have been some of the traditional reasons why people have sought out rural areas for rest, relaxation, and vacations.

Ranchers and farmers have tended to form small close communities which have supported their way of life and provided for mutual support. Depending on their cultural heritage, they have developed and maintained values and attitudes congruent with their way of life. Other groups (e.g., Mexican Americans) have been generally successful in preserving their cultural heritages while attempting to adapt and adjust to changes in United States American society. Others (e.g., Native American groups) have maintained their culture in varying degrees and, in many cases, in relative isolation from the mainstream of U.S. American society.

Much of the history of the United States is concerned with the westward expansion of a civilization that had its beginnings on the eastern shores of the North American continent. The Spaniards were the first men of European origins to penetrate the vast regions between the Rocky Mountains and the Pacific Ocean. As late as the 1820's, very little exploring had been done in the far west. In many cases, the terrain was found to be rough and rugged and resources were scarce in the beginning. Communities were separated by great distances and travel was difficult, at best, by today's standards (Hulse, 1990).

Today, in many areas of the western United States, rural towns and communities may be separated by as much as 100 miles or more. Many of these towns are farm and ranch centers or mining towns. There is often a shortage of physicians, psychiatrists, and psychologists as well as other mental-health-related services and trained personnel. An increase in population in a number of areas within the past 10–15 years has placed a tremendous strain on many local resources. The need for effective community counseling programs in rural areas of the western United States has been increasing. This is at least partially due to stressors placed on old timers and newcomers alike. The rapid growth in some areas is exacerbated by rapidly fluctuating economic changes. As more people enter an area, they tend to overwhelm old timers who quite often are left bewildered and lost in a community which once was theirs. Newcomers have difficulties dealing with scarce or non-existent services and resources as well as a lack of adequate housing. Tensions develop over these areas as well as from a clash of values. There is a need for adequate and effective community counseling centers to address these problem areas.

Human services in any community cover a broad area, In addition to mental health services, such services may include law enforcement, legal services, social services, public health, recreation, youth services, local government, educational services, and services for senior citizens. These services have generally been provided informally or through institutions. When rapid community growth occurs, the size of the local population may increase at a rate which causes people's problems to increase tremendously with a resultant strain on existing community resources.

In areas of rapid development, there tends to be a rapidly developing shortage of adequate and reasonably-priced housing. Rentals become high and crowding develops (Uhlmann, Doherty, and Hill, 1977). Recreation presents other problems. Citizens of rural communities in the west have traditionally engaged in recreational activities such as camping, fishing, and hunting. Newcomers tend to have a different set of interests (e.g., bowling alleys, theaters, swimming pools, and handball courts). Communities which can't provide these types of activities may find newcomers taking advantage of more easily available diversions such as drinking, gambling, and prostitution (Uhlmann, 1977).

Uhlmann (1977) has pointed out a number of significant problem areas in her analysis of the delivery of human services in Wyoming boom towns. Wyoming's boom towns are similar to boom towns in the other western states. Wyoming has a long history of boom-bust cycles – over 100 years worth. The state is currently in a boom cycle in which energy development – e.g., coal, oil, natural gas, wind energy, uranium, trona (sodium carbonate) are providing new workers, development and a surplus in the state budget. However boom cycles always have problems of new people, lack of adequate housing, social services, increases in crime. domestic violence, etc. Wyoming currently has three major boom towns – Gillette and Rock Springs, and western areas around Jackson, Sublette, Pinedale, two of which have had boom-bust cycles since the building of the railroads in the 1800s.

A review of Uhlmann's report points out the potential sources of stress and other mental-health-related problems encountered in western rural communities experiencing rapid growth. She found that mental health problems in rapidly developing communities include an increased incidence of depressed women and a rising rate of alcoholism among males. She also found an increase in family crises and that children and adolescents are at risk for an increased incidence of behavioral disorders and social maladjustments. Newly arrived young adults (18–

26) were found to face problems as a result of few, if any, solid interpersonal relationships. They frequently became involved in drug and alcohol abuse. Uhlmann found that public assistance through social services was drastically reduced and that there was frequently a lack of adequate medical personnel. She found that schools experienced difficulties as a result of a rapid growth in student population. At the high school level, the drop-out rate tended to increase as young people were attracted and drawn off by employment opportunities in the area.

She suggested that law enforcement personnel in rapidly developing communities may have to deal with problems they have not encountered before and may be hampered by inadequate training, low salaries, and a high turnover of personnel. Poor and/or inadequate facilities (e.g., jails, juvenile detention, and foster homes) were seen as making the job of law enforcement more difficult.

Uhlmann suggests that local governments in small rural communities may not have the administrative structure necessary to deal with the new and critical demands placed on them by a rapidly growing population.

In the past, rural communities in the western United States were frequently characterized by a large population of senior citizens. Uhlmann suggests this occurred because young people left the community to seek better employment elsewhere. However, it seems that when a rapid increase in population due to development occurs, this process is partially reversed. Senior citizens may be forced to leave the community due to a rising cost of living. Such a process of demographic change was observed in three Wyoming communities (Uhlmann, Kimble, and Throgmorton, 1976; Uhlmann, Doherty, and Hill, 1977).

Another problem associated with rapid population growth is a sense of a decreasing "quality of life". Rapid growth brings rapid change. Many impacted communities have stressed decline and loss. The negative effects such accounts point out usually include: a speeded-up pace of life; congestion and over- crowding; inflation in prices; fear of change in life style for present residents; lack of activities and sense of belonging for newcomer families; alcoholism and mental health problems (HUD Program Guide, 1976). Increased incidents of severe depression and alienation of both old-timers and new-comers may result in "we–they" conflicts (Miller, 1978).

Traditional agencies and persons who have dealt with the above problem areas may not even exist in such communities. Many of these small rural communities have long been used to everyone taking care of themselves. Existing agencies may find their caseloads overwhelming. Communities which are impacted need help in defining future problems, predicting the magnitude of such problems, and designing and implementing programs and mechanisms to alleviate the problems (Miller, 1978).

Uhlmann (1977) suggests that most of these problems develop because communities don't have the time to develop financial resource bases and local attitudinal support for needed services. She also suggests that problems occur due to the changing composition of local populations. She points out that all of the factors reviewed above bring about increased demands for human services in impacted communities. The remainder of her report focuses on a description of the Wyoming Human Services Project and it focuses on dealing with these problems.

6 | Conclusions: Who are Country Doctors

Rural areas, especially those located in the western United States, present a number of obstacles and lifestyles that are unique. This is generally due to the distances involved, lack of resources often found in more urban environments, a sense of isolation at times, and financial difficulties. Educational resources and opportunities also present challenges. The advent of the internet and computers in more recent times has helped ameliorate some of these. However, these often require financial investments that are often not as easily available as in urban areas. Mental health professionals are even more scarce in rural areas than medical personnel. Professionals in most health and mental health fields face travel over long distances and are often referred to as *circuit riding professionals*

Getting doctors and mental health professionals and keeping them is a constant challenge for rural communities. Working in a small town isn't for everyone. The pace and need for flexibility, in addition to fiscal and lifestyle issues, drive many health and mental health professionals back to the city. For example, "Some physicians find it undesirable to work in a rural setting—it's not 'big-hospital' enough," says Sue Fahey, a certified nurse midwife in Grants Pass, Oregon. "Some physicians thrive on [having] a crisis going on all the time."

For example, Oregon's country doctors, as well as the nurses, dentists, physician assistants and other medical professionals who work in rural communities, are some of the finest health care providers in the state. They serve a large, diverse population with relatively few resources. Although most specialize in general and family practice, country doctors are adept at wearing many different hats and using a wide range of skills to give their patients the best possible care. And because there are so few doctors in small towns, a bad one tends to stick out like a sore thumb and usually doesn't last very long. Similar situations exist in other western rural and frontier states such as Nevada, Wyoming, Montana, Utah, Colorado, and New Mexico.

Who are Country Patients?

The practice of medicine and mental health tends to be done a little differently in the rural west, due in large part due to the type of people that live there. Most live and work independently, as farmers, ranchers, miners, resort workers, and loggers, and spend a lot of time taking care of themselves. As a result, rural health and mental health professionals notice in their communities a tendency for their patients to be stoic and self-reliant, inclined to downplay symptoms and otherwise avoid preventive care.

The best way to treat these kinds of patients, rural health professionals say, is to take time and build relationships with patients/clients. "I get to know people better if I'm slower around them and I give them a chance to tell me what's really on their mind," says Dr. Robert Morrison of Burns, Oregon. "They're rural people and they know how much time it takes to do things."

People who live in rural environs also have different hazards to deal with than people who live in a city. For example, they are more likely to sustain injuries from farm equipment or livestock. They do more driving at high speeds in isolated areas full of mobile wildlife. Some studies indicate higher instances of alcoholism, smoking, and obesity. Heart disease was the number-one cause of death from 1999 to 2001, almost twice as high as cancer-related deaths in similar areas and more than twice as high as deaths from all other sources.

Rural Oregon is poorer than urban Oregon and is also aging faster, as young people graduate from high school and move away. This is a trend seen in most of the rural western states. For example, Halfway, Oregon, saw a 44 percent increase in its 45 to 64-year-old demographic from 1990 to 2002. Many rural adults (some estimate 50 percent) have one or more chronic illnesses. These older patients need more healthcare than ever and rely heavily on Medicare and other government programs to help pay for it.

Economic disincentives are also a factor. Rural medical and mental health professionals tend to get paid less and have a harder time maintaining their practices, which doesn't always jibe with the tens of thousands of dollars in student loans that the average new healthcare and mental health professional has to repay. It may be difficult for a spouse to find work in a small town that supports their own career. The facility in which they work may not be able to afford the newest, most technologically sophisticated equipment. The rural clinic or hospital may have a "tired" appearance with no budget for a remodel. Read more about the challenges of recruiting doctors in the "Choosing a Rural Practice: You Decide" feature in *The Oregon Story* (2010).

http://www.opb.org/programs/oregonstory/countrydocs/decide/launch.html

In some communities, mid-level practitioners such as nurse practitioners and physician assistants are embracing rural practice and picking up where physicians have been leaving off. "Mid-levels," as they are called, have a similar education as physicians, just less of it. For example, a nurse practitioner is a registered nurse who independently provides healthcare in an expanded specialty role, such as family practice or mental health. A physician assistant works under the direction, supervision, and responsibility of a doctor.

Kate Kossler, a family nurse practitioner, was interviewed for the *Hell's Canyon Journal*, which is published in Halfway, Oregon, says that, in some ways, an experienced, rural, mid-level practitioner can have a broader range of skills and be more effective than a new or urban doctor. "A doctor has more training, but a lot depends on experience," she says. "In one day, I could see a car-accident victim, do a well-child exam, treat an elderly patient with diabetes, and see someone with a mental health issue. If a doctor came here and most of his or her prior patient load was kids or just adults, they wouldn't have the same breadth of experience. In a rural clinic, you have to do it all."

Most health and mental health professionals in rural environments are what many refer to as Generalists. In many cases, they may also have little or no experience in dealing with disasters and even certain types of crises or critical incidents. It takes a very special individual with a very special type of dedication to be able to provide health and mental health services in rural environments.

Skills and competencies that are required of disaster mental health professionals are different enough from the typical inpatient/outpatient clinical practice to require more specialized selection and training. When a disaster strikes a community, having a cadre of specially trained mental health professionals who can be quickly mobilized, oriented, and deployed is critical. Most small rural communities often do not have such response capabilities for major disasters. If the impacted area does not have this capacity, mutual aid agreements with those communities that have trained and experienced disaster mental health workers will be helpful in the chaotic times immediately following impact.

Much of the confusion and stress present at the time of disaster impact can be eliminated when a mental health agency and or medical clinic has a core staff pre-designated and trained as a disaster response team. Regular in-service training and participation in disaster exercises in the local jurisdiction can help maintain and fine tune skills. If the resources permit, the team can respond to smaller crises which occur in the jurisdiction. This will provide staff with some first-hand experience they can use when a larger disaster strikes.

Funds for training are hard to come by and sometimes non-existent. Training is considered a necessary and appropriate aspect of the Federal Emergency Management Agency (FEMA) Crisis Counseling programs, both in the Immediate and Regular Programs. Health and Mental health planners and administrators should include realistic training budgets in their grant applications.

Selecting Disaster Mental Health Staff

Rural health and mental health as well as disaster mental health work is not for everyone. They are challenging and rewarding work which requires such professionals to be flexible and socially extroverted. Despite their altruism and sincere desire to help, *not all individuals are well-suited for rural and for disaster work.* Whether designating and training rural and disaster staff, prior to or during a disaster, health and mental health managers should consider several selection issues.

Selection of professional or paraprofessional staff should consider the demographics of the population, including: ethnicity and language, the personality characteristics and social skills of the staff members, and the roles the workers may play in response, treatment, and recovery efforts. Workers who are selected for such work should not be so severely impacted by their work that their responsibilities at home or their emotional reactions will interfere with their responses and interactions within their communities.

Population Demographics

Managers should choose staff that has special skills that match the needs of the population. For example, staff having special expertise working with children and the local schools should be included. If there are many elderly persons in the community, the team should include persons skilled in working with older adults.

Clients and patients must be understood within the context of their ethnic background, cultural viewpoint, life experiences, and values. Those who have limited English-speaking skills may experience difficulty communicating needs and feelings except in their native language. It is important to be sensitive to cultural issues, and services must be provided in ways that are culturally appropriate. Culture in this sense refers to not only ethnic culture, but also the culture of rurality.

It is essential that health and mental health staff be both familiar and comfortable with the culture of the groups they interact with. It is very desirable that they also be fluent in the languages of non-English speaking groups affected. Staff should include individuals who are indigenous to specific cultural and rural groups. If such staff is not immediately available, mutual aid staff with the required ethnic backgrounds and language skills should be recruited from other community agencies or mental health jurisdictions where possible. Indigenous personnel can also be recruited and trained as community peer paraprofessionals.

Personality

The ability to remain focused and to respond appropriately is a key quality for individuals who work in rural areas. Staff must be able to function well in confused, sometimes even chaotic, environments. They must be able to "think on their feet", and have a common-sense, practical, flexible, and often improvisational approach to problem-solving. They must be comfortable with changing situations. They must be able to function with role ambiguity, unclear lines of authority, and a minimum of structure. Many of the most successful health and mental health professionals often perceive these factors as challenges rather than burdens. Initiative and stamina are required, as well as self-awareness and the ability to monitor and manage their own stress.

Professionals need to be able to work cooperatively in a liaison capacity. They need to be aware of and comfortable with value systems and life experiences other than their own. An eagerness to reach out and explore the community to find people needing help, instead of a "wait and treat" attitude, is essential (Farberow and Frederick, 1978). They must enjoy people and not appear lacking in confidence. If the professional is shy or afraid, it will interfere with establishing a connection (DeWolfe, 1992). Staff must be comfortable initiating a conversation in any community setting. In addition, they must be willing and able to "be with" people who may be suffering tragedy and enormous loss without being compelled to try to "fix" the situation.

Health and mental health teams should be multi-disciplinary and multi-skilled. Staff should be experienced in triage, medical first aid, psychological first aid, crisis intervention, and brief treatment. They should have knowledge of crisis, post-traumatic stress, and grief reactions, including disaster psychology. Rural people may be reluctant to come to mental health centers for services. Therefore, staff must be able to provide their services in non-traditional, community-based settings. Prior mental health training and experience are highly recommended. In situations of mutual aid, licensed professionals may need to cross state lines to provide assistance.

Staff should be well-acquainted with the functions and dynamics of the community's human service organizations and agencies (Farberow and Frederick, 1978). They should have experience in consultation and community education. Excellent communication, problem-solving, conflict resolution, and group process skills are needed, in addition to an ability to establish rapport quickly with people from diverse backgrounds.

Managers should pay careful attention to the state's scope of practice laws for various mental health professional disciplines. Individuals providing formal assessment and counseling which fall into the definition of psychotherapy should be appropriately licensed and insured for professional liability.

Qualifications for Professionals

Paraprofessionals can be excellent choices for outreach and community workers. This is especially so if they are familiar with the community and are trusted by its residents. They may already be employed by a mental health, social service, health, or other community-based agency, or they may be recruited from among community residents. Characteristics and qualifications should include the following (Collins and Pancoast, 1976; Farberow and Frederick, 1978; Tierney and Baisden, 1979):

- Possess at least some high school education (to master information and concepts to be taught).
- Are indigenous to the area, if possible.

- Represent a cross section of the community/neighborhood members with regard to age, sex, ethnicity, occupation, length of residence in the community, etc.

- Are motivated to help other people, like people, and have sensitivity and empathy for others.

- Are functioning in a stable, mature, and logical manner.

- Possess sufficient emotional and physical resources and receive sufficient personal rewards as a result and are truly capable of helping.

- Can work cooperatively with others.

- Are able to work with people of other value systems without inflicting their own value systems on others.

- Are able to accept instructions and do not have ready-made, simplistic answers.

- Have an optimistic, yet realistic, view of life, i.e., a "health engendering personality".

- Have a high level of energy to remain active and resourceful in the face of stress.

- Are committed to respecting the confidentiality of others and are not inclined to gossip.

- Have special skills related to unique populations (e.g., children or older adults, particular ethnic groups) or useful to crisis/disaster recovery (e.g., understanding of insurance, building requirements).

- In disasters and/or crises, are able to set personal limits and not become too involved with survivor recovery (e.g., understand the difference between facilitating and empowering survivors as opposed to "taking over" for the survivor).

Circuit Riding the Great Divide: Health and Mental Health in the Frontier Rural Western US – How They Intersect

Major changes in America's general workforce are anticipated between now and the year 2025. Rural people and rural communities face many of the same healthcare issues and challenges confronting the rest of the country—exploding healthcare costs, large numbers of uninsured and underinsured people, an overextended healthcare infrastructure. However, there are numerous unique healthcare issues that face rural people and rural places. Rural America is often viewed and defined by what it lacks. More than 60 percent of rural Americans live in "mental health professional shortage areas". Over 90 percent of all psychologists and psychiatrists, and 80 percent of MSWs, work exclusively in metropolitan areas. More than 65 percent of rural Americans get their mental healthcare from their primary care provider. This series will discuss what rural is, the health and mental health issues faced in rural areas of the western frontier states and other rural areas, identify the problems, resources or lack thereof, some possible solutions, how health and behavioral health interact, and some models to address the future.

Conclusion

This course and each of the chapters and topics presented are offered as an overview and introduction to both the practice of mental health in rural and frontier areas and how to integrate disaster mental health principles and methods into existing systems, organizations, and practices. This course is Part 1 of what will be a series of courses relating to different aspects of mental health and disaster mental health in rural areas and different rural cultures.

The following presents a number of resources and references that hopefully will contribute to a better understanding of rural mental health and disaster mental health. It is not necessarily exhaustive. However, it will be added to and updated in future courses offered in these directions.

Bibliography

Abad, V., Ramos, J. & Boyce, E. (1974). A model for delivery of mental health services to Spanish-speaking minorities. *American Journal of Orthopsychiatry*, 44, 584-595.

Abel, T. (1956). Cultural patterns as they affect psychotherapeutic procedures. *American Journal of Psychotherapy*, 10, 728-740.

Abramowitz, C.V. & Dokecki, P.R. (1977).The politics of clinical judgment: Early empirical returns. *Psychological Bulletin*, 84, 460-476.

Aderibigbe, Yekeen A.; Bloch, Richard M.; Pandurangi, Anand (Jun 2003). Emotional and somatic distress in eastern North Carolina: Help-seeking behaviors. *International Journal of Social Psychiatry*, Vol 49(2), pp. 126-141 .

Aguilera, D.M. & Planchon, L.A. (1995). *The American Psychological Association-California Psychological Association disaster response project: Lessons learned from the past, guidelines for the future.* Professional Psychology: Research

Alexander, A.A., Klein, M., Miller, M. & Workneh, F.(1982). Psychotherapy and the foreign student. In Pedersen, P., Draguns, J.G., Lonner, W.J. & Trimble, J. (Eds.), *Counseling across cultures. (2nd ed.)* Honolulu: University Press of Hawaii.

American Academy of Child and Adolescent Psychiatry. (1998). *Facts for families: Helping*

American Red Cross. (1997). *Emotional health issues for victims*. Arlington, VA: Author.

American Red Cross (1996). Disaster Mental Health Provider's Course (ARC 3076A). *(Manual available to those who take the course)* and Human Services and Mental Health Treatment Similarities and Differences. Washington, DC.

Anderson, Dorothy B. (Apr 1976). An operational framework for working with rural families in crisis. *Journal of Marital & Family Therapy*, Vol 2(2), pp. 145-154.

Apetekar, L. and Boore, J.A. (1990*). The emotional effects of disaster on children*: A review

Austin J, McBride A, Davis H (1989). *Parental attitude and adjustment Research and Practice*, in McCubbin HI, Thompson AI (eds). 43:550-55 1.6. http://www.jcn.sagepub.com/content/12/3/187.full.pdf

Atkinson, D.R., Maruyama, M. & Matsui, S. (1978). Effects of counselor race and counseling approach on Asian American' perceptions of counselor credibility and utility. *Journal of Counseling Psychology*, 25, 76-83.

Author. 1991. (Manual available Project COPE). Washington, D.C.: FEMA Publication.

Banks, G., Berenson, B. & Carkhuff, R. (1967). The effects of counselor race and training upon counseling process with Negro clients in initial interviews. Journal of Clinical Psychology, 23, 70-72.

Banta, Lawrence E. (1991). Major mental illness in two Kenyan outposts. In: Okpaku, Samuel O. (Ed) *Mental health in Africa and the Americas today: A book of conference proceedings*. Nashville, TN, US: Chrisolith Books. pp. 187-193.

Barbopoulos, Anastasia & Clark, James M. (Nov 2003). Practising Psychology in Rural Settings: Issues and Guidelines. *Canadian Psychology*, Vol 44(4), pp. 410-424.

Bartholomew, Kim & Horowitz, Leonard M. (Aug 1991). Attachment styles among young adults: A test of a four-category model. *Journal of Personality & Social Psychology*, Vol. 61(2), pp. 226-244.

Bassuk, Ellen L.; Cote, William (Mar 1983). A network approach to rural psychiatric emergency training. *Hospital & Community Psychiatry*, Vol 34(3), pp. 233-238.

Beare, Paul (Aug 1981). Mainstreaming approach for behaviorally disordered secondary students in a rural school district. *Behavioral Disorders*, Vol 6(4), pp. 209-218.

BellSouth Foundation, the University of Miami, and 7-Dippity, Inc.

Benswanger, Ellen G.; Baider, Lea; Cornely, Paul J. (Spr 1980). Infant death in rural community: Implications for research and intervention. *Journal of Rural Community Psychology*, Vol 1(1), pp. 25-46.

Bertness, Jan E. (Mar 1987). Hazard perception research: A critique and proposal. *Dissertation Abstracts International*, Vol 47(9-A), pp. 3528.

Bertolote, Jose M. & Fleischmann, Alexandra (Jun 2002). "Suicide rates in China, 1995-99": Comment. *Lancet*, Vol 359(9325), pp. 2274.

Bourne, Peter G. (Apr 1974). Approaches to drug abuse prevention and treatment in rural areas. *Journal of Psychedelic Drugs*, Vol 6(2), pp. 285-289.

Bowlby, J. (1982). *Attachment and loss* (Vol. 1). London: The Hogarth Press.

Brady, Kristine Lynn & Caraway, S. Jean (Nov 2002). Home away from home: Factors associated with current functioning in children living in a residential treatment setting. *Child Abuse & Neglect*, Vol 26(11), pp. 1149-1163.

Brandon, Jonathan Henry (May 2000). Working models of self and other in adult attachment and vicarious traumatization. *Dissertation Abstracts International: Section B: The Sciences & Engineering*, Vol 60(10-B), pp. 5219.

Bruner, Jerome S. (Nov-Dec 1990). Culture and human development: A new look. *Human Development*, Vol 33(6). *Special Topic: Jerome Bruner: Construction of a scientist*. pp. 344-355.

Buffalo Creek Flood. (1976). New York: Simon and Schuster.

Bushy, Angeline; Rauh, J. Randall (Apr 1993). The human response to professional litigation in rural practice: Application of Caplan's theory of crisis. *Family & Community Health*, Vol 16(1), pp. 55-66.

Butler, Robert N. (1963). Psychiatric evaluation of the aged. *Geriatrics*, 18(3), pp. 220-232.

Campbell, Lisa Cecilia (Oct 2002). Life stories altered: The effect of clinical depression on reminiscence functions in rural older adults. *Dissertation Abstracts International: Section B: The Sciences & Engineering*, Vol 63(4-B), pp. 2050.

Carlson, E.A. and Sroufe, L.A. (1995). Contribution of attachment theory to developmental.

Carlson, E.B. and Dalenberg, C.J. (2000). A Conceptual Framework for the Impact of Traumatic Experiences In B.A. van der Kolk, A.C., McFarlane, and L. Weisaeth (Eds.). *International Review of Psychiatry,* 6, 141-151.

Carson, David K.; Araquistain, Mary & Ide, Betty (Jun 1994). Stress, strain, and hardiness as predictors of adaptation in farm and ranch families. *Journal of Child & Family Studies,* Vol 3(2), pp. 157-174.

Cassidy, J., Kirsh, S. J., Scolton, K. L., Parke, R.D. (1996). Attachment and Representations of Peer Relationships. Developmental Psychology, 32, 5, 892-904.

Cecchini, Tracy Black (Jun 1998). An interpersonal and cognitive-behavioral approach to childhood depression: A school-based primary prevention study. *Dissertation Abstracts International: Section B: The Sciences & Engineering,* Vol 58(12-B), pp. 6803.

Cecil, Harry F. (Win 1988). Stress: Country Style: Illinois response to farm stress. *Journal of Rural Community Psychology,* Vol 9(2), *Special Issue: Mental health and the crisis of rural America.* pp. 51-60.

Center for Mental Health Services (1993). *Taking Rural Into Account: Report on the National Public Forum.* Washington, D.C.: U.S. Department of Health and Human Services.

Center for Mental Health Services (1994). *Program Guidance: Crisis Counseling and Mental Health Treatment Similarities and Differences.* Washington, D.C.: U.S. Department of Health and Human Services.

Center for Mental Health Services (1996). *Psychosocial Issues for Children and Families in Disasters.* Washington, D.C.: U.S. Department of Health and Human Services.

Center for Mental Health Services.(1994). *Disaster Response and Recovery: A Handbook for Mental Health Professionals.* Washington, D.C. U.S. Department of Health and Human Services; Publication No. (SMA) 94-3010.

Cicchetti, D. & Cohen, D. J. (1995). Perspectives on developmental psychopathology. In D. Cicchetti & D. J. Cohen (Eds.) *Developmental psychopathology, Vol. I: Theory and methods* (pp. 3-22). New York: John Wiley & Sons, Inc.

Cohler, Bertram J. (1993). Aging, morale, and meaning: The nexus of narrative. In: Cole, Thomas R. (Ed); Achenbaum, W. Andrew (Ed). *Voices and visions of aging: Toward a critical gerontology.* New York, NY, US: Springer Publishing Co. pp. 107-133.

Collins, Sean & Long, A. (Aug 2003). Working with the psychological effects of trauma: Consequences for mental health-care workers: A literature review. *Journal of Psychiatric & Mental Health Nursing,* Vol. 10(4), pp. 417-424.

Collomb, H. (1973). L'avenir de la psychiatrie en Afrique. Psychopathologie Africaine, 9, 343-370.

Conger, Katherine Jewsbury; Rueter, Martha A. & Conger, Rand D. (2000). The role of economic pressure in the lives of parents and their adolescents: The Family Stress Model. In: Crockett, Lisa J. (Ed); Silbereisen, Rainer K. (Ed); *Negotiating adolescence in times of social change.* New York, NY, US: Cambridge University Press. pp. 201-223.

Conger, Rand D.; Elder, Glen H. Jr. & Lorenz, Frederick O. (1994). *Families in troubled times: Adapting to change in rural America.* Hawthorne, NY, US: Aldine de Gruyter. xi, 303 pp.

Connery, Hilary Smith (Jan-Feb 2003). Acute symptoms and functional impairment related to September 11 terrorist attacks among rural community outpatients with severe mental illness. *Harvard Review of Psychiatry,* Vol 11(1), pp. 37-42.

Cook, John R. & Tyler, John D. (Sum 1989). Help-seeking attitudes of North Dakota farm couples. *Journal of Rural Community Psychology,* Vol 10(1), pp. 17-28.

Cook, Stephen W. & Heppner, P. Paul (Jan 1997). Coping, control. problem-solving appraisal, and depressive symptoms during a farm crisis. *Journal of Mental Health Counseling,* Vol 19(1), pp. 64-77.

Cook, J. D. & Bickman L. (1989) Social Support and Psychological Symptomatology Following a Natural Disaster. Guidelines for the Future. *Professional Psychology Research and Practice* 26,6, 550-557

Cosario, W.A. (1997). *The sociology of childhood.* Thousand Oaks, CA: Pine Forge

Cowen, Perle Slavik (Dec 2001). Crisis child care: Implications from family interventions. *Journal of the American Psychiatric Nurses Association*, Vol 7(6), pp. 196-203.

Cowen, Perle Slavik (Jul-Sep 1998). Crisis child care: An intervention for at-risk families. *Issues in Comprehensive Pediatric Nursing*, Vol 21(3), pp. 147-158.

Creamer, Terri Lynn (Jan 2002). Secondary trauma and coping processes among disaster mental health workers responding to the September 11th attacks. *Dissertation Abstracts International: Section B: The Sciences & Engineering*, Vol. 63(6-B), pp. 2786.

Crighton, Eric J.; Elliott, Susan J.; van der Meer, Joost (Feb 2003). Impacts of an environmental disaster on psychosocial health and well-being in Karakalpakstan. *Social Science & Medicine*, Vol 56(3), pp. 551-567.

Cunningham, Maddy (Oct 2003). Impact of trauma work on social work clinicians: Empirical findings. ,i>Social Work, Vol 48(4), pp. 451-459.

Dalton, Lisa Ellen (Sep 2001). Secondary traumatic stress and Texas social workers. *Dissertation Abstracts International Section A: Humanities & Social Sciences*, Vol 62(3-A), pp. 1209.

David, K.H. (1976). The use of social learning theory in preventing intercultural adjustment problems. In Pedersen, P., Lonner, W.J. & Draguns, J.G. (Eds.), Counseling across cultures. Honolulu: University of Hawaii Press.

Davis, Helen Miller (Jan 2002). Play and culture: Peer social organizations in three Costa Rican preschools. *Dissertation Abstracts International: Section B: The Sciences & Engineering*, Vol 63(6-B), pp. 3040.

Davis-Brown, Karen & Salamon, Sonya (Oct 1987). Farm families in crisis: An application of stress theory to farm family research. *Family Relations: Journal of Applied Family & Child Studies*, Vol 36(4), *Special Issue: Rural families: Stability and Change*. pp. 368-373.

DeFrain, John & Schroff, Jan A. (1991). Environment and fatherhood: Rural and urban influences. In: Bozett, Frederick W. (Ed); Hanson, Shirley M. H. (Ed); *Fatherhood and families in cultural context*. New York, NY, US: Springer Publishing Co. pp. 162-186.

Denison, John M.(Jan 1971). An unusual social experiment to help youth in crisis (Ankh). Canadian Medical Association Journal, Vol. 104(1), pp. 15-19.

Dimmick, Susan L.; Burgiss, Samuel G.; Robbins, Sherry (Spr 2003). Outcomes of an Integrated Telehealth Network Demonstration Project. *Telemedicine Journal & e-Health, Vol 9(1), Special Issue: Success Stories in Telemedicine: Some Empirical Evidence.* pp. 13-23.

Derosa, Ruth Reed (Dec 1995). Post-traumatic stress disorder and the subjective experience of disaster: The Hamlet fire. *Dissertation Abstracts International: Section B: The Sciences & Engineering*, Vol 56(6-B), pp. 3441. .

Derr, Victoria (Mar-Jun 2002). Children's sense of place in northern New Mexico. *Journal of Environmental Psychology*, Vol 22(1-2), Special Issue: Children and the environment. pp. 125-137.

Derr, Victoria Leigh (May 2002). Voices from the mountains: Children's sense of place in three communities of northern New Mexico. *Dissertation Abstracts International Section A: Humanities & Social Sciences*, Vol 62(10-A), pp. 3454.

Deveraux, G. (1951). Three technical problems in psychotherapy of Plains Indian patients. American Journal of Psychotherapy, 5, 411-423.

Deveraux, G. (1953). Cultural factors in psychoanalytic therapy. Journal of the American Psychoanalytic Association, 1(4), 629-635.

Deveraux, G. (1969). *Reality and the dream: Psychotherapy of a Plains Indian.* Garden City, NY: Doubleday.

DeWolfe, D.J. (2000). *Training manual for disaster mental health workers* (2nd Ed.).

Dinkmeyer, Don & Carlson, Jon (Jan 1990). Guidance in a small school. *School Counselor*, Vol 37(3), pp. 199-203.

Diop, B., Collignon, R. & Gueye, E. (1976). Presentation de l'etude concertee de l'O.M.S. sur les strategies pour l'extension pes soins de sante mentale. Psychopathologie Africaine, 12, 173-188.

Author. Disabilities. The Children of the Flood. Produced by The Farm Disaster: A Guidebook for Teachers. Washington, D.C.: FEMA Disaster: A study of Buffalo Creek. New York: Academic Press, 1981.

Doherty, George W. (Fal 1984). Mental health in a rural area: A program description. *Journal of Rural Community Psychology*, Vol 5(2), pp. 55-63.

Downey, James E. (1978). One year later: Crisis intervention in a rural population: Brief report. *Crisis Intervention*, Vol 9(1), pp. 32-38.

Draguns, J.G. (1975). Resocialization into culture: The complexities of taking a worldwide view of psychotherapy. In Brislin, R.W., Bochner, S. & Lonner, W.J. (Eds.), *Cross-cultural perspectives on learning*. New York: Sage Publications.

Draguns, J.G. (1981). Cross-cultural counseling and psychotherapy: History, issues, current status. In Marsella, A.J. & Pedersen, P.B. (Eds.), *Cross-cultural counseling and psychotherapy*. New York: Pergamon Press.

Dudley-Grant, G. Rita; Mendez, Gloria I. & Zinn, Juliana (Aug 2000). Strategies for anticipating and preventing psychological trauma of hurricanes through community education. *Professional Psychology: Research & Practice*, Vol 31(4), pp. 387-392. .

Duncan, Cynthia M. (1992). *Rural Poverty in America*. New York: Auburn House.

Earls, Felton; Smith, Elizabeth; Reich, Wendy (Jan 1988). Investigating psychopathological consequences of a disaster in children: A pilot study incorporating a structured diagnostic interview. *Journal of the American Academy of Child & Adolescent Psychiatry*, Vol 27(1), pp. 90-95.

Echterling, L. G.; Bradfield, C. and Wylie, M. L. (Sum 1988). Responses of urban and rural ministers to a natural disaster. *Journal of Rural Community Psychology*, Vol 9(1), pp. 36-46.

Echterling, L.G. (1988). An ark of prevention: Preventing school absenteeism after a flood.

Echterling, Lennis G. & Hoschar, Kevin (1989). Using the personal computer in disaster intervention. *Computers in Human Services*, Vol 5(3-4), pp. 157-161.

Eidelson, Roy J.; D'Alessio, Gerard R. & Eidelson, Judy I. (Apr 2003). The impact of September 11 on psychologists. *Professional Psychology: Research & Practice*, Vol 34(2), pp. 144-150.

Elder, Glen H. Jr. & Russell, Stephen T. (2000). Surmounting life's disadvantage. In: Crockett, Lisa J. (Ed); Silbereisen, Rainer K. (Ed); *Negotiating adolescence in times of social change.* New York, NY, US: Cambridge University Press. pp. 17-35.

Elder, Glen H. Jr.; King, Valarie & Conger, Rand D. (1996). Attachment to place and migration prospects: A developmental perspective. *Journal of Research on Adolescence,* Vol 6(4), pp. 397-425.

Elder, Glen H. Jr.; Robertson, Elizabeth B. & Ardelt, Monika (1994). In: Conger, Rand D.; Elder, Glen H. Jr.; *Families under economic pressure. Families in troubled times: Adapting to change in rural America.* Hawthorne, NY, US: Aldine de Gruyter. pp. 79-103.

Erikson, E.H. (1950). Childhood and society. New York: Norton.

Erikson, K.T. (1976). *Everything in its Path: Destruction of Community in the Buffalo Creek Flood.* New York: Simon and Schuster.

Erinosho, O.A. (1976). Lambo's model of psychiatric care. Psychopatgologie Africaine,12, 35-44.

Eyles, John; Taylor, S. Martin & Baxter, Jamie (Jun 1993). The social construction of risk in a rural community: Responses of local residents to the 1990 Hagersville (Ontario) tire fire. *Risk Analysis,* Vol 13 (3), pp. 281-290.

Fabrega, Horacio & Nutini, Hugo (Dec 1994). Tlaxcalan constructions of acute grief. *Culture, Medicine & Psychiatry,* Vol 18(4), pp. 405-431.

Falicki, Zdzislaw; Borowski, Tadeusz; Kalinowski, Antoni (1972). The opinions of rural population on psychic diseases. *Polish Medical Journal,* Vol. 11(1), pp. 213-219. .

Farberow, Norman L. (Fal 1985). Mental health aspects of disaster in smaller communities. *American Journal of Social Psychiatry,* Vol 5(4), pp. 43-55.

Farmer, Val (Apr 1986). Broken heartland. *Psychology Today,* Vol 20(4), pp. 54-57, 60-62.

Federal Emergency Management Agency (1991). *How to Help Children After a Disaster: A Guidebook for Teachers.* Washington, D.C.: FEMA Publication #219.

Federal Emergency Management Agency (1991). *School Intervention Following a Critical Incident. Project COPE.* Washington, D.C.: FEMA Publication #220.

Felner, Robert D (Win 1980). Family stress and organization following parental divorce or death. *Journal of Divorce*, Vol 4(2), pp. 67-76.

Felner, Robert D.; Ginter, Melanie A.; Boike, Mary F. (Apr 1981). Parental death or divorce and the school adjustment of young children. *American Journal of Community Psychology*, Vol 9(2), pp. 181-191.

Ferguson, Stanley B. & Engels, Dennis W. (Mar 1989). American farmers: Workers in transition. *Career Development Quarterly*, Vol 37(3), pp. 240-248.

Fiasche, Angel (1967). Investigation of a chain of suicides in a rural community. *Psychotherapy & Psychosomatics*, 15(1), pp. 20. .

Flynn, B.W. and Nelson, M.E. (1998). Understanding the needs of children following large-scale

Forducey, Pamela G.; Ruwe, William D.; Dawson, Stephen J. (2003). Using telerehabilitation to promote TBI recovery and transfer of knowledge. *NeuroRehabilitation*, Vol 18(2), pp. 103-111.

Forrest, Sandy (Sum 1988). Suicide and the rural adolescent. *Adolescence*, Vol 23(90), pp. 341-347.

Freud, S. (1953). From the history of an infantile neurosis. In J. Strachey (Ed.), *The standard edition of the complete psychological works of Sigmund Freud*, Vol. 17, London: Hogarth.

Friedman, Tatiana Ryk (Mar 2002). The role of empathy in vicarious traumatization. *Dissertation Abstracts International: Section B: The Sciences & Engineering*, Vol 62(8-B), pp. 3799.

Galea, S. (2005). Posttraumatic stress symptoms in children after hurricane Andrew. *Journal of Abnormal* Practice, Vol 31(1) 93-94.

Gamble, Sarah J. (2002). Self-care for bereavement counselors. In: Webb, Nancy Boyd (Ed). *Helping bereaved children: A handbook for practitioners (2nd ed.)*. New York, NY, US: Guilford Press. pp. 346-362.

Gavin, Bea (May 2003). Open space. Some thoughts on moving west. *Psychodynamic Practice: Individuals, groups & organisations*, Vol 9(2), pp. 195-199 .

Gergen, Kenneth J. (1996). Beyond life narratives in the therapeutic encounter. In: Birren, James E. (Ed); Kenyon, Gary M. (Ed). *Aging and biography:*

Explorations in adult development. New York, NY, US: Springer Publishing Co. pp. 205-223.

Ginexi, Elizabeth M.; Weihs, Karen & Simmens, Samuel J. (Aug 2000). Natural disaster and depression: A prospective investigation of reactions to the 1993 Midwest floods. *American Journal of Community Psychology*, Vol 28(4), pp. 495-518.

Giordano, J. & Giordano, G.P. (1976). Ethnicity and community mental health. Community Mental Health Review, 1, No. 3, 4-1`4, 15.

Gist, Richard & Lubin, Bernard (1999). Response To Disaster: Psychosocial, Community, and Ecological Approaches. Brunner-Routledge.

Gleser G.C., Green B.L., Winget C. (1981). *Prolonged Psychosocial Effects of Disaster: A study of Buffalo Creek.* New York: Academic Press.

Glidewell, Reba Sue Ellis (Apr 2001). Burnout, vicarious traumatization, coping styles, and empathy in long-term care nursing personnel. *Dissertation Abstracts International: Section B: The Sciences & Engineering*, Vol 61(9-B), pp. 4982.

Gorgievski-Duijvesteijn, Marjan J. (Apr 1999). Job-involvement and stress in farm-couples; *Gedrag & Gezondheid: Tijdschrift voor Psychologie & Gezondheid*, Vol 27(1-2), pp. 109-117.

Green, B. L.; Korol, M.; and Grace, M. C.; et al. (1991). "Children and Disaster: Age, Gender, and Parental Effects on PTSD Symptoms." *Journal of the American Academy of Child and Adolescent Psychiatry* 30(6):945–951.

Hall, Alan (May 1998). Sustainable agriculture and conservation tillage: Managing the contradictions. *Canadian Review of Sociology & Anthropology*, Vol 35(2), pp. 221-251.

Hanson, R. Karl; Whitman, Robert (Spr 1995). A rural, community action model for the treatment of abusive men. *Canadian Journal of Community Mental Health*, Vol 14(1), pp. 49-59.

Hargrove, David S. (Win 1986). Rural community psychology and the farm foreclosure crisis. *Journal of Rural Community Psychology*, Vol 7(2), Special Issue: Prevention and promotion. pp. 16-26.

Harper, Roy L. (Spr 1984). Crisis Intervention in rural Alaska. *Emotional First Aid: A Journal of Crisis Intervention*, Vol 1(1), pp. 34-38.

Hartsough, Don M. & Myers, Diane Garaventa (1985, reprinted 1987). *Disaster work and mental health: Prevention and control of stress among workers.* Rockville, MD, US: National Institute of Mental Health. v, 149 pp.

Hartup, W.W. (1979). The social worlds of childhood. *American Psychologist,* 34(10), 944-950.

Health and Human Services, 1993. Publication No. (ADM) 83-538, 1983.

Heffron, Edward F. (Apr 1977). Project Outreach: Crisis intervention following natural disaster. *Journal of Community Psychology,* Vol 5(2), pp. 103-111.

Hessen, Erik (Oct 1989). Psykososial stottetjeneste etter en flyulykke: Erfaringer fra en psykiatrisk poliklinikk ved et lokalsykehus. Translated Title: Psychosocial support work after an aircraft accident. *Tidsskrift for Norsk Psykologforening,* Vol 26(10), pp. 696-704. Publisher: Norway: Norsk Psykologforening. Publisher URL: http://www.psykol.no

Higginbotham, H.N. (1976). A conceptual model for the delivery of psychological services in non-western settings. Topics in Culture Learning, 4, 44-52.

Higginbotham, H.N. (1979). Culture and mental health services in developing countries. In A.J. Marsella, Ciborowski, T. & Tharp, R. (Eds.), Perspectives in cross-cultural psychology. New York: Academic Press.

Higginbotham, H.N. (1979). Culture and the delivery of psychological services in developing nations. Transcultural Psychiatric Research Review, 16, 7-27. (a)

Hill, Michele B. (2000). Building sustainable reconciliation in South African communities experiencing witch burnings. *Dissertation Abstracts International: Section B: The Sciences & Engineering,* Vol 60(12-B), pp. 6018.

http://www.aacap.org/web/aacap/facts/factsFam/disaster.htm

http://www.ag.uiuc.edu/~disaster/teacher/teacher.html

http://www.redcross.org/disaster/safety

Hulse, James W. (1990). *Nevada adventure: A history.* University of Nevada Press; 6th edition.

Hutner, Michael & Windle, Charles (Mar 1991). NIMH support of rural mental health. *American Psychologist,* Vol 46(3), pp. 240-243.

Hutton, David Gordon (2003). Patterns and predictors of psychological coping and adjustment among riverbank displacees in an urban environment: A case study of squatters in bangladesh. *Dissertation Abstracts International: Section B: The Sciences & Engineering*, Vol 64(2-B), pp. 966.

Jensen, Gail M. & Royeen, Charlotte B. (May 2002). Improved rural access to care: Dimensions of best practice. *Journal of Interprofessional Care*, Vol 16(2) pp. 117-128.

Jilek-Aal, W. (1978). Native renaissance: The survival and revival of indigenous therapeutic ceremonials among North American Indians. Transcultural Psychiatric Research Review, 15, 117-148.

Johnson, B. B. (Mar-Apr 1987). Sexual abuse prevention: A rural interdisciplinary effort. *Child Welfare*, Vol 66(2), pp. 165-173.

Johnson, Barbara B. (Mar-Apr 1987). Sexual abuse prevention: A rural interdisciplinary effort. *Child Welfare*, Vol 66(2), pp. 165-173.

Jurich, Anthony P.; Russell, Candyce S. (Oct 1987). Family therapy with rural families in a time of farm crisis. *Family Relations: Journal of Applied Family & Child Studies, Vol 36(4), Special Issue: Rural families: Stability and change.* pp. 364-367.

Keating, Norah C. & Munro, Brenda (Apr 1989). Transferring the family farm: Process and implications. *Family Relations: Journal of Applied Family & Child Studies*, Vol 38(2), pp. 215-219.

Keller, Heidi (Sep-Oct 2003). Moving towards consensus on how to characterize culture: Reply to the comments of Catherine Tamis-LeMonda and Kristin Neff. *Human Development*, Vol 46(5), pp. 328-330 .

Kelly, G. (1955). The psychology of personal constructs. New York: Norton.

Kennedy, David Patrick Jr (2003). Gender, culture change, and fertility decline in honduras: An investigation in anthropological demography. *Dissertation Abstracts International Section A: Humanities & Social Sciences*, Vol 64(3-A), pp. 968.

Kennerley, Cati Marsh (Fal 2003). Cultural Negotiations: Puerto Rican Intellectuals in a State-Sponsored Community Education Project, 1948-1968. *Harvard Educational Review*, Vol 73(3), pp. 416-448.

Kim, Sung Eun (Apr 2000). Vicarious traumatization: The impact of therapists of treating trauma clients. *Dissertation Abstracts International: Section B: The Sciences & Engineering*, Vol 60(9-B), pp. 4892.

Kinzel, Audrey & Nanson, Jo (2000). Education and debriefing: Strategies for preventing crises in crisis-line volunteers. *Crisis*, Vol 21(3), pp. 126-134.

Knight, Richard L.(Editor), Gilgert, Wendell (Editor), Marston, Ed (Editor). (2002). Ranching West of the 100th Meridian: Culture, Ecology, and Economics. Island Press.

Korman, M. (1974). National conference on levels and patterns of professional training in psychology: Major themes. American Psychologist, 29, 441-449.

La Greca, A.M. (2001). September 11, 2001 terrorist attacks (Page x), Coral Gables, FL.
www.psy.miami.edu/faculty/alagreca/helping_america_cope.pdf

La Greca, A. M., Silverman, W. S., Vernberg, E. M., & Prinstein, M. J. (1996). Posttraumatic stress symptoms in children after Hurricane Andrew: A prospective study. *Journal of Consulting and Clinical Psychology, 64*, 712-723.

Lamarche, Andre (1960). Rapport de la commission sur l'hygiene mentale du milieu rural. (Report of the commission on rural mental health). *Hygiene Mentale*, 49, pp. 52-74.

Lamb, H. Richard; In: Hales, Robert E. (Ed); Yudofsky, Stuart C. (Ed) (1996). *Public psychiatry and prevention. The American Psychiatric Press synopsis of psychiatry*. Washington, DC, US: American Psychiatric Association. pp. 1323-1341.

Lambo, T. (1962).The importance of cultural factors in psychiatric treatment. Acta Psychiatrica Scandinavica, 38, 176-179.

Lazarus, A.A. (1976). Multimodal Behavior Therapy Springer Publishing Co.

Lazarus, A.A. (1989). *The practice of multimodal therapy: Systematic, comprehensive*

Lazarus, A.A. (2000). Multimodal replenishment. Professional Psychology Research and psychology. In Cicchetti and D. Cohen (Eds.), *Developmental psychopathology: Vol 1*.

Lazarus, A.A. (1976). Multimodal Behavior Therapy. Springer Publishing Co.

Lazarus, A.A. (1989). The practice of multimodal therapy: Systematic, comprehensive, and effective psychotherapy. Johns Hopkins University Press.

Lazarus, A.A. (2000). Multimodal replenishment. Professional Psychology Research and Practice, Vol 31(1) 93-94.

Lazarus, R.S., Opton, E.Jr., Tomita, M. (1966). A cross-cultural study of stress-reaction patterns in Japan. *Journal of Personality & Social Psychology*, 4(6), pp. 622-633. Journal URL: http://www.apa.org/journals/psp.html

Lerias, Doukessa & Byrne, Mitchell K. (Aug 2003). Vicarious traumatization: symptoms and predictors. *Stress & Health: Journal of the International Society for the Investigation of Stress*, Vol 19(3), pp. 129-138.

Linley, P. Alex; Joseph, Stephen & Cooper, Rachel (Oct 2003). Positive and Negative Changes Following Vicarious Exposure to the September 11 Terrorist Attacks. *Journal of Traumatic Stress*, Vol 16(5), pp. 481-485.

Lobao, L. & Meyer, K.(Dec 1995). Economic decline, gender, and labor flexibility in family-based enterprises: Midwestern farming in the 1980s. *Social Forces*, Vol 74(2), pp. 575-608.

Loeb, E. & Dvorak, J. (1987). Farm families. *Family Therapy Collections*, Vol 22, pp. 97-109.

Lombas, T.M. (Jun 2002). A naturalistic exploration of stress and coping among rural law enforcement officers: Implications for the counseling profession. *Dissertation Abstracts International Section A: Humanities & Social Sciences*, Vol 62(11-A), pp. 3701.

Lowe, A.J. (Jul 2002). On vicarious traumatization: The relationship between trauma, quality of attachment, and defensive style in the emergency room. *Dissertation Abstracts International: Section B: The Sciences & Engineering*, Vol 63(1-B), pp. 535.

Luabe J. and S.A. Murphy (1985). *Perspectives on Disaster Recovery*. Norwalk, CT.: Prentice-Hall.

Lugris, V.M. (May 2001). Vicarious traumatization in therapists: Contributing factors, PTSD symptomatology, and cognitive distortions. *Dissertation Abstracts International: Section B: The Sciences & Engineering*, Vol 61(10-B), pp. 5571.

Lybeck-Brown, J.C. (2003). Vicarious traumatization of psychotherapists: Implications for theory, training, and practice. *Dissertation Abstracts International: Section B: The Sciences & Engineering*, Vol 63(9-B), pp. 4377.

Lystad, M. (1985). Special programs for children. *Children Today,* 14(1), 13-17.

Lystad, M. (1984). *At Home in America: as seen through its books for children.* Cambridge: Schenkman Publishing Company.

Madakasira, S. O'Brien, K.F. (May 1987). Acute posttraumatic stress disorder in victims of a natural disaster. *Journal of Nervous & Mental Disease*, Vol 175(5), pp. 286-290.

Main, M. (1996). Introduction to the special section on attachment and psychopathology: 2. Overview of the field of attachment. *Journal of Consulting and Clinical Psychology*, 64(2), 237-243. Retrieved from http://www.ncbi.nlm.nih.gov/pubmed/8871407

Maltais, D.; Lachance, L. & Brassard, A. (2002). Difficultes et effets a-6 long terme d'une catastrophe en milieu rural: Etude combinant les approches qualitative et quantitative. = A qualitative and quantitiative study of the long-term psychological effects of a natural disaster on a rural community. *Revue Quebecoise de Psychologie*, Vol 23(3), pp. 197-217.

Mandic, N. & Mihaljevic, Z.V. (Dec 1993). Psychologic state of displaced persons from East Slavonia. *Socijalna Psihijatrija*, Vol 21(3-4), pp. 121-135.

Marshall, C.D. (May 1971). The indigenous nurse as community crisis intervener. *Seminars in Psychiatry*, Vol. 3(2), pp. 264-270.

Martinez-Brawley, E.E. & Blundall, J. (Jul 1991). Whom shall we help? Farm families' beliefs and attitudes about need and services. *Social Work*, Vol 36(4), pp. 315-321.

Mash, E.J. and Barkley. R.A. (1993a). Washington, DC: American Psychiatric Press. Green, BL (1993a). *Journal of the American Academy of Child Psychiatry*, 25, 346-356.

McAdams, Dan P. (1993). *The stories we live by: Personal myths and the making of the self.* New York, NY, US: William Morrow & Co, Inc. 336 pp .

McClelland, David C. & Atkinson, J.W. (2000). *Achievement Motive* Irvington Pub.

McDowell, Christopher (2002). Involuntary resettlement, impoverishment risks, and sustainable livelihoods. *Australasian Journal of Disaster and Trauma Studies*, Vol 6(2), pp. [np].

McGowan, Alicen-J. (Mar-Apr 2002). While Waiting for the Other Shoe. *Forensic Examiner*, Vol 11(3-4), pp. 38-39.

McInnes, Rita (Dec 2000). Landed gender: Rural couples caught between traditional and contemporary roles. *Australian & New Zealand Journal of Family Therapy*, Vol 21(4), *Special Issue: Innovative and contextual approaches to human problems.* pp. 191-200.

McLean, Sara; Wade, Tracey D. & Encel, Jason S. (Oct 2003). The Contribution of Therapist Beliefs to Psychological Distress in Therapists: An Investigation of Vicarious Traumatization, Burnout and Symptoms of Avoidance and Intrusion. *Behavioural & Cognitive Psychotherapy*, Vol 31(4), pp. 417-428.

McRee, Christine; Corder, Billie; Deitz, Susan (Win 1985-1986). Short term psychiatric intervention with children and families in a tornado disaster area. *Psychiatric Forum*, Vol 13(2), pp. 86-90.

Mendel, W,M. (1972). Comparative psychotherapy. International Journal of Psychoanalytic Psychotherapy, 1(4), 117-126.

Mermelstein, Joanne & Sundet, Paul (Win 1988). Factors influencing the decision to innovate: The future of community responsive programming. *Journal of Rural Community Psychology*, Vol 9(2), *Special Issue: Mental health and the crisis of rural America.* pp. 61-75.

Mermelstein, Joanne S. (Oct 1987). Criteria of rural mental health Directors in adopting farm crisis programming innovation. *Dissertation Abstracts International*, Vol 48(4-A), pp. 1013-1014.

Miller, Thomas W. & Veltkamp, Lane J. (1988). Child sexual abuse: The abusing family in rural America. *International Journal of Family Psychiatry*, Vol 9(3), pp. 259-275.

Mitchell, J.T. & Everly, G.S., Jr. (1993). Critical incident stress debriefing (CISD): An operations manual for the prevention of traumatic stress among emergency services and disaster workers. Ellicott City, MD: Chevron.

Miura, M. & Usa, S. (1970). A psychotherapy of neurosis: Morita therapy. Psychologia, 13, 18-34.

Moosman, Jennifer L. (May 2002). Vicarious traumatization: The effects of empathy and trait arousability. *Dissertation Abstracts International: Section B: The Sciences & Engineering*, Vol 62(10-B), pp. 4796.

Morris, Jerry A. (1997). The rural psychologist in the hospital emergency room. In: Morris, Jerry A. (Ed) *Practicing psychology in rural settings: Hospital privileges and collaborative care.* Washington, DC, US: American Psychological Association. pp. 81-96.

National Institute of Mental Health (1983). *Training Manual for Human Service Workers in Major Disasters.* Washington, D.C., U.S. Department of Health and Human Services; Publication No. (ADM) 83-538.

Neese, Jane B.; Abraham, Ivo L.; Buckwalter, Kathleen C. (Feb 1999). Utilization of mental health services among rural elderly. *Archives of Psychiatric Nursing*, Vol 13(1), pp. 30-40.

Neff, Kristin (Sep-Oct 2003). Understanding how universal goals of independence and interdependence are manifested within particular cultural contexts. *Human Development*, Vol 46(5), pp. 312-318.

Neff, Kristin (Sep-Oct 2003). Understanding how universal goals of independence and interdependence are manifested within particular cultural contexts. *Human Development*, Vol 46(5), pp. 312-318.

Neki, J.S. (1973). Guru-chepa relationship: The possibility of a therapeutic paradigm. American Journal of Orthopsychiatry, 43, 755-766.

Norris, Fran H.; Phifer, James F. & Kaniasty, Krzysztof (1994). Individual and community reactions to the Kentucky floods: Findings from a longitudinal study of older adults. In: Ursano, Robert J. (Ed); McCaughey, Brian G.(Ed) *Individual and community responses to trauma and disaster: The structure of human chaos.* New York, NY, US: Cambridge University Press. pp. 378-400.

Oakes, Margaret Grace (Dec 1998). Emotional reactions to the trauma of war: A field study of rural El Salvador. *Dissertation Abstracts International Section A: Humanities & Social Sciences*, Vol 59(6-A), pp. 2188.

ODochartaigh Disaster Mental Health Bookstore (2011). http://www.angelfire.com/biz/odochartaigh/searchbooks.html Accessed February 1, 2011.

Oetting, E. R.; Cole, C. W. & Adams, R. (1969). Problems in program evaluation: A ministers' workshop. *Mental Hygiene*, 53(2), pp. 214-217.

Critical incident stress debriefing: Bereavement support in schools. (1994). *Clinical Child Psychology*, 22, 470-484. *International Journal of Mental Health*, 10(2), 77-90.

Olson, Kenneth R. & Schellenberg, Richard P. (Oct 1986). Farm stressors. *American Journal of Community Psychology*, Vol 14(5), *Special Issue: Rural mental health*. pp. 555-569.

Pasternak, Alan Gary (Jan 2002). The lost soldier: A phenomenological study of trauma in noncombat soldiers in the Vietnam war. *Dissertation Abstracts International: Section B: The Sciences & Engineering*, Vol 62(9-B), pp. 4230.

Patrick, V. & Patrick, W. K. (Mar 1981). Cyclone '78 in Sir Lanka: The mental health trail. *British Journal of Psychiatry*, Vol 138, pp. 210-216.

Paulsen, Jane (Sum 1988). Crisis, culture, and response. *Journal of Rural Community Psychology*, Vol 9(1), pp. 5-11.

Paulsen, Julie (Sum 1988). A service response to a culture in crisis. *Journal of Rural Community Psychology*, Vol 9(1), pp. 16-22.

Paynter, Robert (Aug-Oct 2002). Time in the valley: Narratives about rural New England. *Current Anthropology*, Vol 43(Suppl), *Special Issue: Repertoires of timekeeping in anthropology*. pp. S85-S101.

Pearlman, Laurie Anne & Mac Ian, Paula S. (Dec 1995). Vicarious traumatization: An empirical study of the effects of trauma work on trauma therapists. *Professional Psychology: Research & Practice*, Vol 26(6), pp. 558-565.

Pedersen, P. (1976). The cultural inclusiveness of counseling. In Pedersen, P., Draguns, J.G., Lonner, W.J. & Trimble, J. (Eds.), Counseling across cultures. 2nd ed Honolulu: University Press of Hawaii.

Pedersen, P., Lonner, W.J. & Draguns, J.G. (Eds.) (1976). Counseling across cultures. Honolulu: University Press of Hawaii.

Peeks, Barbara (Dec 1989). School-based intervention for farm families in transition. *Elementary School Guidance & Counseling*, Vol 24(2), pp 128-134.

Peeks, Barbara (May 1989). Farm families in crisis: The school counselor's role. *School Counselor*, Vol 36(5), pp. 384-388.

Peltzer, Karl (Oct 1999). Posttraumatic stress symptoms in a population of rural children in South Africa. *Psychological Reports*, Vol 85(2), pp. 646-650.

Peoples, U.Y. & Dell, D.M. (1975). Black and white student preferences for counselor roles. Journal of Counseling Psychology, 22, 529-534.

Perry, Helen Swick; Perry, Stewart E. (1959). *The schoolhouse disasters: Family and community as determinants of the child's response to disaster.* Washington, DC, US : National Academy of Sciences. viii, 66 pp.

Phillips, Michael R.; Li, Xianyun & Zhang, Yanping (Jul 2002). "Suicide rates in China, 1995-99": Erratum. *Lancet*, Vol 360(9329), pp. 344.

Phipps, Andrew B.; Byrne, Mitchell K. (Aug 2003). Brief interventions for secondary trauma: review and recommendations. *Stress & Health: Journal of the International Society for the Investigation of Stress* Vol 19(3), pp. 139-147.

Pierce, Roger Clarke (Aug 2000). Secondary trauma from working with Vietnam veterans. *Dissertation Abstracts International: Section B: The Sciences & Engineering*, Vol 61(2-B), pp. 1093.

Pinter, E. (1969). Wohlstandfluchtlinge. Eine sozialpsychiatrische studie an ungarischen Fluchtlingen in der Schweiz. *Bibliotheca Psychiatrica et Neurologica*, No. 138.

Pinto, Regina Maria (2003). The impact of secondary traumatic stress on novice and expert counselors with and without a history of trauma. *Dissertation Abstracts International Section A: Humanities & Social Sciences*, Vol 63(9-A), pp. 3117.

Plunkett, Scott W.; Henry, Carolyn S.; Knaub & Patricia K. (Spr 1999). Family stressor events, family coping, and adolescent adaptation in farm and ranch families. *Adolescence*, Vol 34(133), pp. 147-168.

Presty, Sharon Katharine (Jul 1996). Psychological sequelae of battered women residing in rural community shelters. *Dissertation Abstracts International: Section B: The Sciences & Engineering*, Vol 57(1-B), pp. 0707.

Prince, R.H. (1976). *Psychotherapy as the manipulation of endogenous healing mechanisms: A transcultural survey.* Transcultural Psychiatric Research Review,13, 115-134.

Prince, R.H. (1980). Variations in psychotherapeutic experience. In H.C. Triandis & J.G. Draguns (Eds.), *Handbook of cross-cultural psychology.* Vol. 6. Psychopathology. Boston: Allyn & Bacon.

Priya, Kumar Ravi (Jan,Jul,& Nov 2002). Suffering and healing among the survivors of Bhuj earthquake. *Psychological Studies*, Vol 47(1-3), pp. 106-112.

Project COPE (1995). Final Report, Northridge Earthquake Crisis Counseling Assistance and Training Regular Program. Ventura County, California.

Project HELP (1994). Flood Crisis Counseling Assistance and Training Program. Wisconsin, 1994. Project Rainbow, Final Report, Flood Crisis Counseling Assistance and Training Regular Program. Missouri.

Project Recovery (1994). Final Report, Flood Crisis Counseling Assistance and Training Regular Program. Illinois.

Provenzo, Eugene F. Jr. & Fradd, Sandra H. (1995). *Hurricane andrew, the public schools and the rebuilding of community.* SUNY.

Pynoos, R.S., Steinberg, A.M., & Goenjian, A. (1996). Traumatic stress in childhood and adolescence: Recent developments and current controversies. In B. A. van der Kolk & A. C. McFarlane (Eds.), *Traumatic Stress: The Effects of Overwhelming Experience on Mind, Body, and Society* (pp. 331–358). New York: Guilford Press

Ragland, John D. & Berman, Alan L. (1990-1991). Farm crisis and suicide: Dying on the vine? *Omega: Journal of Death & Dying*, Vol 22(3), pp. 173-185.

Rajouria, S. (Jan 2002). The natural context of mother-toddler play interactions in a rural Nepali community. *Dissertation Abstracts International Section A: Humanities & Social Sciences*, Vol 63(6-A), pp. 2124 .

Ramirez-Ferrero, E.E. (Apr 2002). Troubled fields: Men, emotions and the Oklahoma farm crisis, 1992--1994. *Dissertation Abstracts International Section A: Humanities & Social Sciences*, Vol 62(9-A), pp. 3097.

Reardon, D.C. (Jun 2002). "Suicide rates in China, 1995-99": Comment. *Lancet*, Vol 359(9325), pp. 2274.

Regehr, Cheryl (Fal 2001). Crisis debriefing groups for emergency responders: Reviewing the evidence. *Brief Treatment & Crisis Intervention*, Vol. 1(2), pp. 87-100.

Reich, Wendy & Earls, Felton (Dec 1987). Rules for making psychiatric diagnoses in children on the basis of multiple sources of information: Preliminary strategies. *Journal of Abnormal Child Psychology*, Vol 15(4), pp. 601-616.

Rettig, Kathryn D.; Danes, Sharon M. & Bauer, Jean W. (May 1991). Family life quality: Theory and assessment in economically stressed farm families. *Social Indicators Research*, Vol 24(3), pp. 269-299.

Reynolds, D.K. (1976). Morita psychotherapy. Berkeley: University of California Press, 1976.

Ricci, Michael A.; Caputo, Michael & Amour, Judith (Spr 2003). Telemedicine Reduces Discrepancies in Rural Trauma Care. *Telemedicine Journal & e-Health*, Vol 9(1), *Special Issue: Success Stories in Telemedicine: Some Empirical Evidence.* pp. 3-11.

Ritz, Sandra Ellen (May 1997). Survivor humor in disasters: Implications for public health training and practice. *Dissertation Abstracts International: Section B: The Sciences & Engineering*, Vol 57(11-B), pp. 6878.

Rogers, Kim Lacy (1994). Trauma redeemed: The narrative construction of social violence. In: McMahan, Eva M. (Ed) & Rogers, Kim Lacy (Ed); *Interactive oral history interviewing*. Hillsdale, NJ, England: Lawrence Erlbaum Associates, Inc. pp. 31-46.

Rose-Gold, Marc S. (Nov 1991). Intervention strategies for counseling at-risk adolescents in rural school districts. *School Counselor*, Vol 39(2), pp. 122-126.

Rosenblatt, Paul C. (1990). *Farming is in our blood: Farm families in economic crisis*. Ames, IA, US : Iowa State University Press . ix, 187 pp.

Ruiz, P. & Langrod, J. (1976). Psychiatrists and spiritual healers: Partners in community mental health. In J. Westermeyer (Ed.), Anthropology and mental health: Setting a new course. The Hague: Mouton.

Ruiz, R.A. & Padilla, A.M. (1977). Counseling Latinos. Personnel and Guidance Journal, 55, 401-408.

Saakvitne, Karen W. and Pearlman, Laurie Anne. (1995). A Video Series on: Vicarious Traumatization. Online: Accessed February 1, 2011 - http://www.cavalcadeproductions.com/vicarious-traumatization.html

Sabin-Farrell, Rachel & Turpin, Graham (May 2003). Vicarious traumatization: Implications for the mental health of health workers? *Clinical Psychology Review*, Vol 23(3), *Special Issue: Post Traumatic Stress Disorder*. pp. 449-480.

Saylor, C.F. (1988). *Children and Disasters*. New York: NY Plenum Press.

Schafer, Roy (1992). *Retelling a life: Narration and dialogue in psychoanalysis.* New York, NY, US : Basic Books, Inc . xvii, 328 pp.

http://www.ag.uiuc.edu/~disaster/teacher/teacher.html Retrieved February 27, 2002.

Schulman, Michael D. & Armstrong, Paula S. (Aug 1989). The farm crisis: An analysis of social psychological distress among North Carolina farm operators. *American Journal of Community Psychology*, Vol 17(4), pp. 423-441.

Schulman, Michael D. & Armstrong, Paula S. (Sep 1990). Perceived stress, social support and survival: North Carolina farm operators and the farm crisis. *Journal of Sociology & Social Welfare*, Vol 17(3), pp. 3-22.

Seebold, Andrew (Sum 2003). Responding To A Murder/Suicide At A Rural Junior High School. *International Journal of Emergency Mental Health*, Vol 5(3), pp. 153-159 .

Selye, Hans (1956). *The stress of life.* 324 pp.

Seward, G. (1956). *Psychotherapy and culture conflict.* New York: Ronald Press.

Sharan, Pratap; Chaudhary, Geeta; Kavathekar, Surabhi A. (Apr 1996). Preliminary report of psychiatric disorders in survivors of a severe earthquake. *American Journal of Psychiatry*, Vol 153(4), pp. 556-558 .

Shore, James H.; Vollmer, William M. & Tatum, Ellie L. (Nov 1989). Community patterns of posttraumatic stress disorders. *Journal of Nervous & Mental Disease*, Vol 177(11), pp. 681-685.

Shows, W. Derek (Fal 1974). A sleeping epidemic among first-grade children: Crisis intervention. *Community Mental Health Journal*, Vol 10(3), pp. 332-336.

Shybut, James E. (1978). One year later: Crisis intervention in a rural population: Brief report. *Crisis Intervention*, Vol 9(1), pp. 32-38.

Shybut, John (Spr 1982). Use of paraprofessionals in enhancing mental health service delivery in rural settings. *Journal of Rural Community Psychology*, Vol 3(1), pp. 59-64.

Silver, Thelma; Goldstein, Howard (Jun 1992). A collaborative model of a county crisis intervention team: The Lake County experience. *Community Mental Health Journal*, Vol 28(3), pp. 249-256.

Slovak, Karen & Singer, Mark (Aug 2001). Gun violence exposure and trauma among rural youth. *Violence & Victims*, Vol 16(4), *Special Issue: Developmental Perspectives on Violence and Victimization.* pp. 389-400.

Slovak, Karen (May 2002). Gun violence and children: Factors related to exposure and trauma. *Health & Social Work*, Vol 27(2), pp. 104-112.

Slovak, Karen Lynne (Mar 2000). The mental health consequences of violence exposure: An exploration of youth in a rural setting. *Dissertation Abstracts International Section A: Humanities & Social Sciences*, Vol 60(8-A), pp. 3138.

Slovak, Karen; Singer, Mark I. (Feb 2002). Children and violence: Findings and implications from a rural community. *Child & Adolescent Social Work Journal*, Vol 19(1), pp. 35-56.

Smith, E.J. (1977). Counseling Black individuals: Some stereotypes. Personnel and Guidance Journal, 55, 390-396.

Smith, G. A.; Thompson, J. D. & Shields, B. J. (Apr 1997). Evaluation of a model for improving emergency medical and trauma services for children in rural areas. *Annals of Emergency Medicine*, Vol 29(4), pp. 504-510.

Snustad, Diane G.; Thompson-Heisterman, Anita A.; Neese, Jane B. (1993). *Clinical Gerontologist* Mental health outreach to rural elderly: Service delivery to a forgotten risk group. Vol 14(1), Special Issue: The forgotten aged: Ethnic, psychiatric, and societal minorities. pp. 95-111.

Solomon, Susan D. & Smith, Elizabeth M. (1994). Social support and perceived control as moderators of responses to dioxin and flood exposure. In: Ursano, Robert J. (Ed); McCaughey, Brian G. (Ed) *Individual and community responses to trauma and disaster: The structure of human chaos.* New York, NY, US: Cambridge University Press. pp. 179-200.

Speilberger, Charles D.; Bale, Ronald M. (Dec 1970). State and trait anxiety in student naval aviators. Bucky, Steven F. *USN AMRL*, No. 1125.

Speir, A. H. (1999). *Disaster response and recovery: A handbook for mental health professionals* (Draft Rev. Ed.). Rockville, MD: Center for Mental Health Services.

State of Illinois Department of Mental Health and Developmental Disabilities (1994). *The Children of the Flood.* Produced by The Farm Resource Center, Videotape.

Stein, Howard F. (Spr 1984). Sittin' tight and bustin' loose: Contradiction and conflict in midwestern masculinity and the psychohistory of America. *Journal of Psychohistory*, Vol 11(4), pp. 501-512.

Strauss, Anselm & Corbin, Juliet (1998). *Basics of qualitative research: Techniques and procedures for developing grounded theory (2nd ed.).* Thousand Oaks, CA, US: Sage Publications, Inc. xiii, 312 pp. [Authored Book]

Strauss, Anselm & Corbin, Juliet M. (1990). *Basics of qualitative research: Grounded theory procedures and techniques.* Thousand Oaks, CA, US: Sage Publications, Inc. 270 pp. [Authored Book]

Strauss, Anselm; Corbin, Juliet (1994). Grounded theory methodology: An overview. In: Denzin, Norman K. (Ed); Lincoln, Yvonna S. (Ed). Handbook of qualitative research. Thousand Oaks, CA, US: Sage Publications, Inc. pp. 273-285. Taplitz-Levy, Beth Dana (Jan 2002). Phoenix falling: The collapse of a collaborative research project. *Dissertation Abstracts International: Section B: The Sciences & Engineering*, Vol 63(6-B), pp. 3071.

Sue, D.W. & Sue, S. (1972). Counseling Chinese-Americans. Personnel and Guidance Journal, 50, 637-644.

Sue, D.W. (1977). Counseling the culturally different: A conceptual analysis. Personnel and Guidance Journal, 55, 422-425.

Sue, S. & McKinney, H. (1975). Asian-Americans in the community mental health care system. American Journal of Orthopsychiatry, 45, 111-118.

Sundet, Paul; Mermelstein, Joanne (1996). Predictors of rural community survival after natural disaster: Implications for social work practice. *Journal of Social Service Research*, Vol 22(1-2), pp. 57-70.

Sutton, John M. Jr. & Pearson, Richard (Apr 2002). The practice of school counseling in rural and small town schools. *Professional School Counseling*, Vol 5(4), pp. 266-276.

Swisher, Raymond R.; Elder, Glen H. Jr. & Lorenz, Frederick O. (Mar 1998). The long arm of the farm: How an occupation structures exposure and vulnerability to stressors across role domains. *Journal of Health & Social Behavior*, Vol 39(1), pp. 72-89.

Szapocznik, J., Scopetta, M.A., Arandale, M.A. & Kurtines, W. (1978). Cuban value structure: Treatment implications. Journal of Consulting and Clinical Psychology, 46, 961-970.

Taft, R. (1977). Coping with unfamiliar environments. in Warren, N. (Ed.), Studies of cross-cultural psychology. Vol. 1. London: Academic Press.

Tanaka-Matsumi, J. (1979). Cultural factors and social influence techniques in Naikan therapy: A Japanese self-observation method. Psychotherapy: Theory, Research and Practice, 16, 385-390.

Taplitz-Levy, Beth Dana (Jan 2002). Phoenix falling: The collapse of a collaborative research project. *Dissertation Abstracts International: Section B: The Sciences & Engineering*, Vol 63(6-B), pp. 3071.

Thompson, Elizabeth A.; McCubbin, Hamilton I. (Oct 1987). Farm families in crisis: An overview of resources. *Family Relations: Journal of Applied Family & Child Studies*, Vol 36(4), *Special Issue: Rural families: Stability and change.* pp. 461-467.

Thurber, Steven (Oct 1977). Natural disaster and the dimensionality of the I-E scale. *Journal of Social Psychology*, Vol 103(1), pp. 159-160.

Torrey, E.F. (1972a). The mind game: Witchdoctors and psychiatrists. New York: Emerson Hall.

Torrey, E.F. (a972). What western psychotherapists can learn from witchdoctors. American Journal of Orthopsychiatry, 42 69-76b.

Tseng, W.S. & Hsu, J. (1979). Culture and psychotherapy. In Marsella, A.J., Tharp, R.G. & Ciborowski, T.J. (Eds.), Perspectives on cross-cultural psychology. New York: Academic Press.

Uhlmann, J.M. (1977). Wyoming Human Services Project Report.

Uhlmann, Doherty, R. and Hill, R. (1977). Wyoming Human Services Project Report.

Uhlmann, Kimble and Throgmorton (1976). Wyoming Human Services Project Report.

University of Illinois at Urbana-Champaign. (1998). *Children, stress, and natural disasters: School activities for children.* Urbana-Champaign, IL: Author

Van Hook, Mary P. (May 1987). Harvest of despair: Using the ABCX model for farm families in crisis. *Social Casework*, Vol 68(5), pp. 273-278.

Van Hook, Mary P. (Win 1990). The Iowa farm crisis: Perceptions, interpretations, and family patterns. *New Directions for Child Development*, No 46, pp. 71-86.

Veenhoven, R. et al. (1994). *Correlates of happiness; 7838 findings from 603 studies in 69 nations 1911-1994* RISBO Studies in Social and Cultural Transformation. Rotterdam: Erasmus University Netherlands (3 volumes).

Vernberg, E.M., LaGreca, A.M., Silverman, W.K. and Prinstein, M.J. (1996). Prediction of

Vogel, J. and Vernberg, E.M. (1993). Children's psychological response to disaster. *Journal*

Vontress, C.E. (1969). Cultural barriers in the counseling relationship. Personnel and Guidance Journal, 48, 11-17.

Vontress, C.E. (1970). Counseling Blacks. Personnel and Guidance Journal, 48, 713-719.

Wagenfeld, Morton O. (Win 1988). Rural mental health and community psychology in the post community mental health era: An overview and introduction to the special issue. *Journal of Rural Community Psychology*, Vol 9(2), *Special Issue: Mental health and the crisis of rural America.* pp. 5-12.

Walker, James L. & Walker, Lilly J. (Jan 1988). Self-reported stress symptoms in farmers. *Journal of Clinical Psychology*, Vol 44(1), pp. 10-16.

Wallace, Julia; O'Hara, Michael W. (Aug 1992). Increases in depressive symptomatology in the rural elderly: Results from a cross-sectional and longitudinal study. *Journal of Abnormal Psychology*, Vol 101(3), pp. 398-404.

Wang, Xiangdong; Gao, Lan; Zhang, Huabiao (Aug 2000). Post-earthquake quality of life and psychological well-being: Longitudinal evaluation in a rural community sample in northern China. *Psychiatry & Clinical Neurosciences*, Vol 54(4), pp. 427-433.

Wang, Xiangdong; Zhang, Huabiao; Naotaka, Shinfuku (1999). Assessment of the quality of life in a rural community affected by an earthquake. *Chinese Mental Health Journal*, Vol 13(1), pp. 24-27.

Weaks, K.A. (Apr 2000). Effects of treating trauma survivors: Vicarious traumatization and style of coping. *Dissertation Abstracts International: Section B: The Sciences & Engineering*, Vol 60(9-B), pp. 4915.

Webb, Dianne B. (Jan 1989). PBB: An environmental contaminant in Michigan. *Journal of Community Psychology*, Vol 17(1), pp. 30-46.

Webster, J.D. (1995). Adult age differences in reminiscence functions. In: Haight, Barbara K. (Ed); Webster, Jeffrey Dean (Ed). *The art and science of reminiscing: Theory, research, methods, and applications*. Philadelphia, PA, US: Taylor & Francis. pp. 89-102.

Webster, J.D. (Sep 1993). Construction and validation of the Reminiscence Functions Scale. *Journals of Gerontology*, Vol 48(5), pp. P256-P262.

Webster, J.D. (Spr 1997). Attachment style and well-being in elderly adults: A preliminary investigation. *Canadian Journal on Aging*, Vol 16(1), pp. 101-111.

Webster, J.D. (Spr 1999). World views and narrative gerontology: Situating reminiscence behavior within a lifespan perspective. *Journal of Aging Studies*, Vol 13(1). *Special Issue: Narrative gerontology*. pp. 29-42.

Webster, J.D.; McCall, M.E. (Jan 1999). Reminiscence functions across adulthood: A replication and extension. *Journal of Adult Development*, Vol 6(1). *Special Issue: Aging and autobiographical memory*. pp. 73-85.

Weidman, H. (1975). Concepts as strategies for change. Psychiatric Annals, 5, 312-314.

Wendt, S.& Cheers, B. (Jun 2002). Impacts of rural culture on domestic violence. *Rural Social Work*, Vol 7(1), pp. 22-32.

Wendt, Sarah; Taylor, Judy & Kennedy, Marie (Dec 2002). Rural domestic violence: Moving towards feminist poststructural understandings. *Rural Social Work*, Vol 7(2), pp. 26-30.

Wertz, Christina Ann (Apr 2001). Vicarious traumatization: The relationship of absorption, emotional empathy and exposure to traumatized clients to ptsd symptom-like behavior in therapists. *Dissertation Abstracts International: Section B: The Sciences & Engineering*, Vol 61(9-B), pp. 5013.

Weyer, Sharon M.; Hustey, Victoria R. & Rathbun, Lesley (Apr 2003). A look into the Amish culture: What should we learn? *Journal of Transcultural Nursing*, Vol 14(2), pp. 139-145

Whitsel, Bradley Christian (Mar 1999). Escape to the mountains: A case study of the Church Universal and Triumphant. *Dissertation Abstracts International Section A: Humanities & Social Sciences*, Vol 59(9-A), pp. 3634.

Willson, E. A. (1928). Education and occupation of farm reared children. *Quarterly Journal of the University of North Dakota*, 18, pp. 361-373.

Wise, Paula S.; Smead, Valerie S. (Fal 1985). Establishing the need for crisis intervention in rural schools. *Emotional First Aid: A Journal of Crisis Intervention*, Vol 2(3), pp. 3-9.

Wittkower, E.D. & Warnes, H. (1974). Cultural aspects of psychotherapy. *American Journal of Psychotherapy*, 28, 566-573.

Wrenn, G.C (1962). *The culturally encapsulated counselor*. Harvard Educational Review, 32, 444-449.

Yule, W. and Canterbury, R. (1994). *The treatment of post traumatic stress disorder in children*

Zargar, Akbar; Najarian, Bahman; Roger, Derek (1993). Settlement reconstruction and psychological recovery in Iran. In: Wilson, John Preston (Ed); Raphael, Beverley (Ed). *International handbook of traumatic stress syndromes*. New York, NY, US: Plenum Press. pp. 979-988.

Zimmerman, Toni Schindler (Apr 1994). Family ranching and farming: A consensus management model to improve family functioning and decrease work stress. *Family Relations: Interdisciplinary Journal of Applied Family Studies* Vol 43(2), pp. 125-131.

Appendix: Resource Materials

Saakvitne, K. W., & Pearlman, L. A. (1996). *Transforming the pain: A workbook on vicarious traumatization*. New York: W.W. Norton & Company.

American Red Cross. Disaster Mental Health Provider's Course (ARC 3076A). April, 1991. (Manual available to those who take the course)

Disaster Mental Health References and Resources

- Rocky Mountain Region Disaster Mental Health – Conference Proceedings –
  http://www.rmrinstitute.org/books.html

- Related Articles
  http://www.rmrinstitute.org/articles.html

- Related Journals
  http://www.rmrinstitute.org/journals.html

- Natural Hazards Observer
  http://www.colorado.edu/hazards/o/archives/2008/Jul08/JulyObserverweb.pdf

- CISM Annotated Links
  http://www.rmrinstitute.org/cismlinks.html

- Gulf War Syndrome
  http://www.angelfire.com/biz/odoc/gulf.html

- Wildland Fire Information
  http://www.angelfire.com/biz3/news/wildfires.html

- Rocky Mountain Region Disaster Mental Health Institute
  http://www.rmrinstitute.org/rocky.html

INTERVIEWS and Reviews

Below are interviews for books by online and radio book reviewers in Austin, TX (Inside Scoop Live) and others. Radio interviews are mp3 available through the following links for those interested:

"From Crisis to Recovery: Strategic Planning for Response, Resilience, and Recovery" Interview is at: http://www.insidescooplive.com/author-pages/Doherty-George-reading-interview.html

Sources of Assistance and Information

Government

Federal Emergency Management Agency (FEMA)

FEMA coordinates with other state and Federal agencies to respond to Presidentially declared disasters. It provides disaster assistance for individuals, businesses (through the Small Business Administration), and communities under the Stafford Act.

Federal Emergency Management Agency
Human Services Division
500 C Street SW
Washington, D.C. 20472
(202) 646-3929
Website www.fema.gov

Center for Mental Health Services (CMHS), Substance Abuse and Mental Health Services Administration (SAMHSA)

Through an interagency agreement with FEMA, CMHS provides consultation and technical assistance on the Crisis Counseling Assistance and Training Program. Publications and videotapes on disaster human response are readily available through SAMHSA's National Mental Health Information Center.

Center for Mental Health Services
Emergency Services and Disaster Relief Branch
5600 Fishers Lane, Room 17C-20
Rockville, MD 20857
(301) 443-4735
FAX (301) 443-8040

CMHS Clearinghouse
SAMHSA's National Mental Health Information Center
P.O. Box 42557
Washington, D.C. 20015

Toll-Free Information Line 1-800-789-2647
FAX 240-221-4295
(TDD) 866-889-2647
Website www.mentalhealth.samhsa.gov

National

American Red Cross (ARC) ARC has chapters in most large cities and a state chapter in each capital city. Every local Red Cross chapter is charged with readiness and response responsibilities in collaboration with its disaster partners. Disaster services include preparedness training, community education, mitigation, and response. They help families with immediate basic needs (food, clothing, shelter) as well as supportive services and longer term interventions. Contact the local chapter for assistance or the state chapter in your capital city.

American Red Cross
431 18th Street N.W.
Washington, D.C. 20006
(202) 737-8300 General Information
(703) 206-7460 Disaster Services
Website www.redcross.org

Professional Organizations

Many professional organizations have gathered resources and information at national and state levels. Some may have established a formal network of professionals qualified to serve as consultants or volunteers. Helpful organizations include but are not limited to the following:

American Psychological Association (APA)
750 First Street, N.E.
Washington, D.C. 20002-4242
(202) 336-5898

National Association of Social Workers (NASW)
750 First St. N.E., Suite 700
Washington, D.C. 20002-4241
(202) 408-8600
1-800-638-8799

National Rural Health Association
1320 19th Street, N.W., Suite 350
Washington, D.C. 20036-1610
(202) 232-6200

National Association for Rural Mental Health
P.O. Box 570
Wood River, IL 62095
(618) 251-0589

State and Local

Department of Mental Health

Contact the state agency responsible for mental health services. There may be a state disaster mental health coordinator already designated to manage the Crisis Counseling Program. This main office will be located in your state's capital city.

Emergency Services

This is the lead agency delegated by the governor to carry the day-to-day emergency management responsibilities. Contact the Office of Emergency Services in your capital city.

Universities and Medical Universities

Academic practitioners with general training in stress, coping, and counseling often express interest in offering assistance. Caution is advised to assure that disaster survivors are treated appropriately, and not enlisted into a research study or given treatments designed for traditional psychiatric disasters. Undergraduate and graduate students are usually very interested in serving as crisis counselors. Contact your local university's department of psychiatry, psychology, or social work.

Religious Organizations

Churches, synagogues, and interfaith organizations provide a valuable resource for finding and serving disaster survivors. Often, they are the most productive and rapid responders for immediate basic needs. Most denominations have some kind of disaster relief program. Contact the district office for major denominations in your area.

Media

Television, radio, and newspapers should provide a listing of available resources and supports in major disasters.

Volunteer Organizations

National Volunteer Organizations Active in Disasters (NVOAD)

NVOAD has made disaster response a priority. Member organizations provide effective service and avoid duplicating services by coordinating them before a disaster strikes. Member organizations include:

- Adventist Community Services (ACS)
- American Relay League, Inc. (ARL)
- American Red Cross (ARC)
- AMURT (Ananda Marga Universal Relief Team)
- Catholic Charities USA (CC)
- Christian Disaster Response, A.E.C.C.G.C.
- Christian Reformed World Relief Committee (CRWRC)
- Church of the Brethren (CB)
- Church World Service (CWS)
- The Episcopal Church (EC)
- Friends Disaster Service (FDS)
- Inter-Lutheran Disaster Response (ILDR)
- Mennonite Disaster Service (MDS)
- Nazarene Disaster Response (NDR)
- The Phoenix Society (PS)
- The Points of Light Foundation (PLF)
- Presbyterian Church, USA (PC)
- REACT International, Inc.(REACT)
- The Salvation Army (SA)
- Second Harvest National Network of Food Banks (SHNNFB)

- Society of St. Vincent de Paul (SSVP)
- Southern Baptist Convention (SBC)
- United Methodist Church Committee of Relief (UMCOR)
- Volunteers of America (VOA)
- World Vision (WV)

Glossary of Terms

The following is an abridged version of the Center for Mental Health Services glossary, explaining terms that are often used in Disaster Mental Health responses. You may encounter these (and other) words and acronyms while reviewing literature on disaster response and recovery. Familiarity with these terms as well as the functions they fulfill is important for those who propose to work as Disaster Mental Health Responders.

Center for Mental Health Services (CMHS)

CMHS is a center within the Substance Abuse Mental Health Services Administration (SAMHSA) and located in Rockville, Maryland. CMHS advises the Federal Emergency Management Agency (FEMA) on disaster mental health. SAMHSA is part of the Department of Health and Human Services (DHHS).

Community Mental Health Center (CMHC)

The CMHC is the administrative agent that contracts with the state department of mental health to provide mental health services to clients in a specified service area, usually covering one or more counties.

Crisis Counseling Assistance and Training Program

The Crisis Counseling Assistance and Training Program (commonly referred to as the Crisis Counseling Program) is funded by the Federal Emergency Management Agency (FEMA) through the Robert T. Stafford Disaster Relief and Emergency Assistance Act (Public Law 93-288 as amended by Public Law 100-707). Services offered by the Crisis Counseling Program involve direct interventions, as well as crisis counseling to individuals and groups impacted by a major disaster or its aftermath. Educational activities and public information on disaster mental health issues are another component of the Crisis Counseling Program. In addition, disaster mental health consultation and training are also provided.

The Crisis Counseling Program includes two separate funding mechanisms: Immediate Services (IS) and Regular Services (RS). States must apply for the IS within fourteen calendar days after the Presidential disaster declaration. FEMA may fund the IS for up to sixty-days after the declaration date. The RS is designed to provide up to nine months of crisis counseling services, community outreach, and consultation and education services to people affected by the disaster. Although states must submit an application for RS funds to FEMA within sixty-days of the disaster declaration, the RS funding is awarded through CMHS based on a formal review of the grant application.

Director, Human Services Division

Located at FEMA Headquarters in Washington, D.C., this person approves or disapproves a request for Regular Service funding for crisis counseling under section 416 of the Stafford Act.

Disaster Recovery Manager (DRM)

This person is appointed to exercise the authority of the FEMA Regional Director for a particular emergency or major disaster.

Disaster Field Office (DFO)

When a disaster strikes and FEMA is activated to respond, a DFO is opened, generally near the disaster site. Many functions are performed and programs run from this office. The DFO is a joint Federal/State operation.

Emergency Operations Center (EOC)

This is the nerve center of disaster recovery operation and is usually under the jurisdiction of the local government. It may be located in or near government offices to allow access to records and resources. The EOC is usually designed to be self-sufficient for a reasonable amount of time with provisions for electricity, water, sewage disposal, ventilation, and security. The major functions of the EOC are information management, situation assessment, and resource allocation.

Emergency Management Institute (EMI)

EMI is located at 16825 South Seton Avenue, Emmitsburg, Maryland 21727, 1-800-238-3358. EMI serves as the national focal point of the Federal Emergency Management Agency for the development and delivery of emergency management training to enhance capabilities of Federal, state, and local government officials, volunteer organizations, and the private sector. EMI programs focus on minimizing the impact of disaster on the American public. The curricula are structured to meet the needs of this diverse audience with an emphasis on how various elements work together in emergencies to save lives and protect property.

Emergency Services and Disaster Relief Branch (ESDRB)

This branch is within the Division of Program Development, Special Populations and Projects of CMHS and provides disaster mental health technical assistance to FEMA and the state mental health authority on the crisis counseling program. A project officer is assigned to the state for the regular service grant and monitors programming and expenditures. ESDRB is located at 5600 Fishers Lane, Room 17C-20, Parklawn Building, Rockville, Maryland, 20857. The telephone number is (301) 443-4735. FAX 301-443-8040.

Federal Emergency Management Agency (FEMA)

FEMA is the lead Federal agency in disaster response and recovery. The Stafford Act provides the authority for the Federal government to respond to disasters and emergencies in order to provide assistance to save lives and protect public health, safety, and property. FEMA provides funding for crisis counseling grants to state mental health departments following Presidentially declared disasters.

Federal Coordinating Officer (FCO)

This person is appointed by the President to coordinate Federal assistance in an emergency or major disaster. The FCO acts as the President's representative on-site during a disaster recovery operation. The positions of Disaster Recovery Manager (DRM) and FCO are usually held by the same person.

Gatekeepers

Gatekeepers are people within the community who can provide access to target populations and are part of the community support system. Examples include teachers, clergy, school counselors, physicians, healthcare workers, welfare workers, funeral directors, and others.

Governor's Authorized Representative (GAR)

This person is appointed by the Governor and has the authority to execute all necessary documents for disaster assistance on behalf of the state. Often the GAR and the State Coordinating Officer (SCO) are the same person.

Human Services (HS)/Individual Assistance (IA)

FEMA disaster programs and services include assistance for individual disaster survivors/victims and their families. Major HS programs include: Disaster Unemployment Assistance, Individual and Family Grant Program, Disaster Housing Program, Cora Brown Fund, and Crisis Counseling Assistance and Training. HS programs were called IA programs prior to 1992. Some state offices of emergency management still refer to IA programs.

Immediate Services (IS)

The IS grant is for the initial crisis counseling response. Although programming may be continued through the RS Grant, funding is considered separate and comes from FEMA. IS funding may be approved in response to a state request for up to sixty-days from the date of the Presidential Declaration or until an RS is funded. Reimbursement for eligible expenses incurred between the date of the disaster occurrence and the disaster declaration may be provided through the immediate services program.

Key Informants

Key informants are people within the community who, through their regular contact with local residents, can provide information on who is impacted by the disaster. In rural areas, key informants include healthcare personnel such as physicians, nurses and pharmacists; ministers, pastors and clergy members; beauticians and barbers; and senior center personnel.

National Association of State Mental Health Program Directors (NASMHPD)

The directors of state departments of mental health comprise this organization located at 66 Canal Center Plaza, Suite 302, Alexandria, VA 22314 (703) 739-9333.

National Voluntary Organizations Active in Disasters (NVOAD)

NVOAD is a group of voluntary organizations that have made disaster response a priority. State VOADs also exist and can direct local organizations and governments to resources within their area. If unable to determine the state VOAD coordinator, contact the national VOAD coordinator at (301) 270-6782.

Project Officer (PO)

The PO is the person representing CMHS to monitor the crisis counseling project, provide consultation, technical assistance and guidance, and be the contact point within the Department of Health and Human Services for the mental health services provided following a disaster.

Public Assistance (PA)

FEMA funds programs and services available to communities impacted by disasters. This is the "bricks and mortar" response such as debris removal and road and bridge reconstruction.

Regional Director (RD)

FEMA is divided into ten regions, each run by a regional director. The RD has authority to approve or disapprove immediate services funding requests for the Crisis Counseling Assistance and Training Program.

Regular Services (RS)

The RS grant funds recovery crisis counseling services following a disaster. RS can be funded for up to nine months. An extension can be requested due to documented extreme need for three months beyond the initial nine-month period. Program and funds are monitored by CMHS.

Robert T. Stafford Disaster Relief and Emergency Assistance Act (Stafford Act)

The Stafford Act is the legislation that enables Federal emergency response and services to be provided following a disaster. Section 416 authorizes the President to provide Crisis Counseling Assistance and Training for disaster victims following Presidentially declared disasters.

Substance Abuse Mental Health Services Administration (SAMHSA)

The Department of Health and Human Services (DHHS) houses SAMHSA, which is divided into three centers: the Center for Mental Health Services (CMHS), the Center for Substance Abuse Prevention (CSAP) and the Center for Substance Abuse Treatment (CSAT). CMHS provides the technical assistance to FEMA for the Crisis Counseling Program.

State Coordinating Officer (SCO)

The SCO is the person appointed by the Governor to work in cooperation with the Federal Coordinating Officer. Often, the SCO and the GAR are the same person.

Unmet Needs Committees (UNC)

Often, local disaster services groups form an unmet needs committee to review survivors'/victims' needs, pool resources, and ensure non-duplication of services. Committees meet on a regular basis. Crisis counseling representatives ensure that the disaster mental health needs are met not only for the survivors but for committee members as well.

About the Author

George Doherty resides in Laramie, WY where he founded the Rocky Mountain Region Disaster Mental Health Institute, Inc. He is currently employed as the President/CEO of this organization and also serves as Clinical Coordinator of the Snowy Range Critical Incident Stress Management Team.

He has been involved with disaster relief since 1995, serving as a Disaster Mental Health Specialist with such incidents as the UP train wreck in Laramie, Hurricane Fran in North Carolina, the Cincinnati floods in Falmouth, KY and Tropical Storm Allison in Southeast Texas. He served as Supervisor for Disaster Mental Health for flash floods in Ft. Collins, and spent a month as the Red Cross Disaster Mental Health Coordinator for western Puerto Rico in the aftermath of Hurricane George.

He has also published numerous articles in disaster mental health and traumatic stress publications and served as Guest Editor for two Special Editions of the journal *Traumatology* (1999 & 2004).

He served as an officer in the US Air Force and was an OTS instructor, squadron commander and other positions. Additionally, he served 11 years involved in Air Search & Rescue with Civil Air Patrol (US Air Force Auxiliary) in WY as Squadron Commander, Deputy Wing Commander, Air Operations Officer, and Master Observer. He is a Certified Instructor with the Wyoming Peace Officers Standards and Training (POST).

He has extensive experience conducting CISM debriefings with first responders and others and is a member of a national crisis care network, providing assistance to companies and other organizations following critical incidents involving sudden deaths and similar traumatic events.

He is a Licensed Professional Counselor in private practice and has been an adjunct instructor for a number of colleges, including Northern Nevada Community College and the University of Wyoming. Organizational memberships include the American Counseling Association, Voting Associate Member of the American Psychological Association, American Academy of Experts in Traumatic Stress (AETS), Association of Traumatic Stress Specialists (ATSS), Traumatic

Incident Reduction Association (TIRA), Certificate of Specialized Training in the field of Mass Disaster and Terrorism, Wyoming Department of Health Hospital Emergency Preparedness Advisory Committee; Research Advisor and Research Fellow: American Biographical Institute (ABI), Editorial Advisory Board Member and Book Reviewer: PsyCritiques (*APA Journal*), Life Member of the Air Force Association, Life Member of the Military Officers Association of America, Member American Legion, Life Member: Pennsylvania State University Alumni Association, Alumni Admissions Volunteer - Pennsylvania State University.

Publications include: Crisis *Intervention Training for Disaster Workers: An Introduction.*; Editor and contributor for the *Proceedings of Rocky Mountain Region Disaster Mental Health Conferences* (2005, 2006, 2007, 2008). Served as Guest Editor for Special issues of the journal *Traumatology* on Disaster Mental Health (1999) and Crises in Rural America (2004); Cross-cultural Counseling in Disaster Settings. - *Australasian Journal of Disaster and Trauma Studies* (1999). Published reviews include: Understanding Oslo in Troubled Times; Responders to September 11, 2001: Counseling: Innovative Responses to 9/11 Firefighters, Families, and Communities; Genocide: A Human Condition?; Stress Management, Wellness and Organizational Health; Leadership Competency and Conflict; Leadership: Lessons from the Ancient World - all in PsyCritiques. Conference Director for annual Rocky Mountain Disaster Mental Health Conferences 1999 - present.

Additional past positions include: Masters Level Psychologist – Rural Clinics (State of Nevada), 1980 – 1986; Veterans Counselor (VA Contract) – 1980-1986, NV; Counselor – pre-delinquent children and families – CORA Services (Philadelphia, PA).1972-1975; Program Coordinator – Community Action Programs (EOAC, Office of Economic Opportunity – Waco/McLennan County, TX) 1968-1971.

Current Courses/Workshops he teaches include:

- Crisis Intervention In Disasters: Training For Workers - An Introduction - 12 CEU
- CISM: Individual Crisis Intervention And Peer Support
- CISM: Group Crisis Intervention
- CISM: Advanced Group Crisis Intervention
- CISM: Strategic Response to Crisis (Capstone Course)
- Return To Equilibrium: Disaster Mental Health- 4 CEU

- Return To Equilibrium: Returning Military And Families - 8 CEU
- From Crisis to Recovery: Strategic Planning for Response, Resilience and Recovery - 12 CEU

Email: rockymountain@mail2emergency.com and rmrinstitute@wyoming.usa.com

About the Rocky Mountain Region Disaster Mental Health Institute

Mission:

The Rocky Mountain Region Disaster Mental Health Institute is an independent, nonprofit, 501(c)(3) corporation whose mission is to promote the development and application of practice, research, and training in disaster mental health, Critical Incident Stress Management, traumatology and other emergency response interventions and the promotion of community awareness, resilience and recovery. This includes hazards vulnerability and mitigation research, planning and training for first responders, mental health professionals, chaplains and related personnel.

Purpose:

The purpose of the Institute is to provide a forum for presentation of research results, education, training and consultation in Disaster Mental Health Services (DMHS) and Critical Incident Stress Management (CISD/CISM), advances in delivery of DMHS and CISD/CISM, discussion and sharing of information, ideas and plans, development of a DMHS and CISD/CISM research and service delivery network, presentation of Continuing Education training for mental health professionals, first responders and chaplains, training for newly recruited DMHS and CISD/CISM volunteers and first responders, and publication of program proceedings and papers as appropriate for dissemination to DMHS and CISD/CISM professionals and first responders locally, regionally and nationally.

Significance:

Mental Health Services before, during and following disasters, critical incidents, crises, and terrorist activities are becoming an integral part of disaster and critical incident preparedness, mitigation, response, and follow-up. Disaster Mental Health Services is a relatively new field which has expanded significantly within the past ten years. Critical Incident Stress Debriefing and Critical Incident Stress

Management have been around since the early 1980s. In order to continue to grow and meet identified needs, both will require continued development as well as focused research and training. Research will help identify how Mental Health Services can best be utilized as well as how relevant changes need to be made in practice. Networking and sharing experiences can also help develop resources.

The long-term goal includes training emergency Disaster Mental Health teams and CISM teams to conduct interventions for corporations, states, municipalities and rural communities in the Rocky Mountain region and to evaluate their effectiveness in reducing the effects of trauma on first responders and others as well as affected communities and organizations.

Who Should Attend

The conference is a must experience for anyone working in the fields of: emergency medical services and trauma units, crisis intervention, mental health, traumatic stress, emergency services, disaster mental health, military, National Guard & Reserve, schools, law enforcement, firefighters, chaplains and other first responders.

Certificates of Attendance

All conference delegates will be provided with Certificates of Attendance. Each presentation will be listed on the reverse with the number of contact hours. It is the responsibility of the delegate to have each presenter sign off on their certificate. Your Certificate of Attendance will be printed with your name exactly as it appears on your Registration form. Please make sure that you print it clearly. A small fee of $5.00 will be assessed to make and mail a duplicate certificate. If you register late or onsite, your certificate will be printed and mailed approximately 3 weeks post-conference.

Rocky Mountain Region Disaster Mental Health Institute
Po Box 786
Laramie, WY 82073-0786

http://www.rmrinstitute.org/rocky.html
email: rockymountain@mail2emergency.com
Phone: 307-399-4818

The Rocky Mountain Region Disaster Mental Health Institute is a 501(c)3 Non-profit Organization.

RMRDMHI BOARD OF DIRECTORS

President of Institute

George W. Doherty, MS, LPC
Laramie, WY

Board Members

David Smith Laramie, WY	**Chaplain Bob Rudichar** Campbell County Memorial Hospital Gillette, WY
Thomas Mitchell, LPC Torrington, WY	**David King** Campbell County Emergency Manager Gillette, WY
Sgt. Randy Hanson Rock Springs PD Rock Springs, WY	**Stewart Anderson** Casper/Natrona County Emergency Manager Casper, WY
Theresa Simpson Casper/Natrona County Deputy Emergency Manager Casper, WY	**Daniel R. Bogart, MA** Evanston, WY

Index

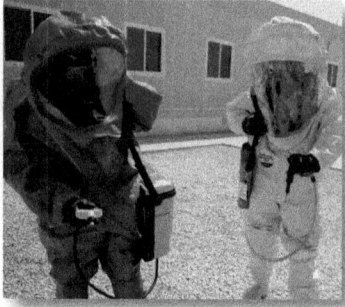

From Crisis to Recovery
Strategic Planning for Response, Resilience, and Recovery

GEORGE W. DOHERTY, MS, LPC

Crises Happen... Will *You* Be Ready?

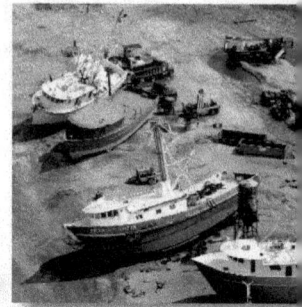

Crises affect people on many different levels, including psychological well-being. The 2004/2009 tsunamis, hurricanes Rita and Katrina, and wars in Iraq and Afghanistan are among events continuing to affect millions of lives daily. Potential events like Avian and Swine Flu pandemics, global warming/climate change, and threats of spreading unrest in the Middle East are concerns weighing heavily on all. Planning and coordination are important components of responses to crises, disasters, and critical incidents.

Resilience, recovery from crises, community preparation, learning from past experience, and strategically planning for future events are all activities involving education, training, and time of first responders, behavioral health professionals, chaplains and others. Additional response variables include cultural knowledge and sensitivity. We need to respond appropriately within a culture not our own, whether locally, nationally, or internationally. The purpose of a behavioral health plan is to ensure efficient, coordinated, and effective responses to behavioral health needs of affected populations during times of disasters and other critical incidents.

Readers of this book will:

- Learn how the community and individuals respond to recover from disasters.
- Identify activities in preparing for, responding to, and recovering from disasters.
- Perform strategic planning and explain how it is helpful in mitigating and responding to disasters, critical incidents and other crises.
- Understand the mental health services provided to people affected by disasters, critical incidents and other crises.
- Identify and explain how disaster mental health professionals are affected by responding to disasters, critical incidents and other crises.
- Understand the stages of disaster recovery and how resilience affects each stage.
- Learn the signs and symptoms of disaster-induced stress and emotional trauma and how resilience mitigates outcomes.
- Discover the meaning of "Return to Equilibrium" and explain its role in the recovery process following a disaster or critical incident.

"Learning from the past and planning for the future"

ISBN-13: 978-1-61599-015-3
Pages: 280
Trim: 7.44 x 9.69" Paperback
List: $29.95
Available at Amazon.com and other fine bookstores.

PO Box 786
Laramie, WY 82073-0786
Phone: 307-399-4818
www.RMRinstitute.org

Crisis Intervention Training for Disaster Workers

George W. Doherty, MS, LPC

This book provides information about training for mental health professionals and first responders who work with victims of disaster related stress and trauma. It helps prepare them to relate with disaster victims and co-workers. Warning signs and symptoms are explored together with stages, strategies and interventions for recovery.

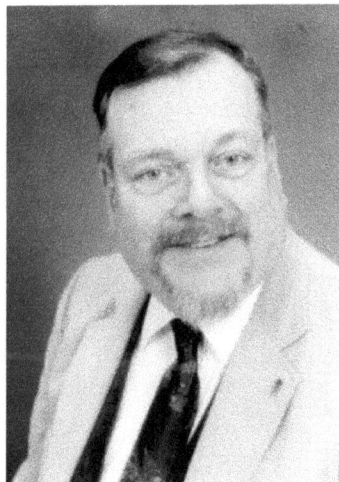

The book will introduce you to disasters, the community response, the roles of first responders, Disaster Mental Health Services and Critical Incident Stress Management (CISM) responders and teams. It provides a brief overview of these and their roles in responding to the needs of both victims and disaster workers. The role of CISM is presented and discussed both for disasters and other critical incidents. This includes discussion about war, terrorism and follow-up responses by mental health professionals. The book is designed to help readers identify appropriate methods for activating Disaster Mental Health Crisis Intervention Teams for disaster mental health services for victims, co-workers, and self.

The content includes general theory and models of Disaster Mental Health, CISM, crisis intervention techniques commonly used in these situations, supportive research, and practice of approaches used in responding to the victims, workers and communities affected by disasters, critical incidents and terrorism threats and events.

"Provides a breadth and depth of knowledge as well as practical tools for beginner to expert. Should be required reading for all disaster responders, and, especially, mental health professionals considering disaster work."
　　—Bruce L. Andrews, MS, LPC (ARC Disaster Mental Provider/Instructor)

"This text serves as a wonderful adjunct and lead into the discipline of CISM. It provides a brief survey of disaster mental health and disaster mental health services."
　　—Thomas Mitchell, LPC

ISBN-13: 978-1-932690-42-2
Pages: 288
Trim: 7.44 x 9.69" Paperback
List: $29.95

Available at Amazon.com and other fine bookstores.

Rocky Mountain
Disaster Mental Health Institute
Press

"Learning from the past and planning for the future"

RMRInstitute.org